Epilepsy and Migraine

Epilepsy and Migraine

Editors:
Dominique Parain
Renzo Guerrini
Dale Hesdorffer
Philippe Ryvlin

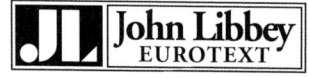

ISBN: 978-2-7420-0654-0
Current Problems in Epilepsy, vol. 22
ISSN: 0950-4591

Éditions John Libbey Eurotext
127, avenue de la République
92120 Montrouge, France
Tél. : 33 (0)1 46 73 06 60
e-mail : contact@jle.com
http://www.jle.com

Editor: Anne Chevalier

John Libbey Eurotext
42-46 High Street
Esher, Surrey
KT10 9KY
United Kingdom

© 2009 John Libbey Eurotext. All rights reserved.

It is prohibited to reproduce this work or any part of it without authorisation of the publisher or of the Centre Français d'Exploitation du Droit de Copie (CFC), 20, rue des Grands-Augustins, 75006 Paris.

List of contributors

Carmen Barba, Pediatric Neurology Unit and Laboratories, Children's Hospital A. Meyer, University of Florence, Firenze, Italy

Christelle Créac'h, Saint-Étienne Pain Center, Saint-Étienne, France

Jean-Christophe Cuvellier, Department of Child Neurology, Pediatric Clinic, University Hospital, Lille, France

Geneviève Demarquay, Department of Neurology, Hôpital de la Croix-Rousse, Lyon, France

Anne Donnet, Department of Neurosurgery, La Timone Hospital, Marseille France

Gilles Géraud, Department of Neurology, University Hospital, Toulouse, France

Évelyne Guégan-Massardier, Department of Neurology, University Hospital, Rouen, France

Renzo Guerrini, Pediatric Neurology Unit and Laboratories, Children's Hospital A. Meyer, University of Florence, Firenze, Italy

Lucie Guyant-Maréchal, Department of Neurology, University Hospital, Rouen, France

Dale C. Hesdorffer, Gertrude H. Sergievsky Center and Department of Epidemiology, Columbia University, New York, USA

Axel Lebas, Department of Neurophysiology, University Hospital, Rouen, France

Dominique Parain, Department of Neurophysiology, University Hospital, Rouen, France

Sylvain Rheims, Neurology Hospital and CTRS-Inserm IDÉE (Childhood and Adolescence Epilepsy Institute), Lyon, France

Philippe Ryvlin, Neurology Hospital and CTRS-Inserm IDÉE (Childhood and Adolescence Epilepsy Institute), Lyon, France

Louis Vallée, Department of Child Neurology, Pediatric Clinic, University Hospital, Lille Cedex, France

Contents

- Comorbidity of epilepsy and migraine: epidemiological considerations 1
  Dale C. Hesdorffer

- Migraine's pathophysiological mechanisms 21
  Gilles Géraud

- What the epileptologist has to know about the International Headache Society classification of migraine 33
  Anne Donnet

- Epilepsy and migraine: a disorder of hyperexcitability? 41
  Geneviève Demarquay, Christelle Créac'h, Sylvain Rheims, Philippe Ryvlin

- Epilepsy and migraine: clinical phenomenology and co-occurrence of symptoms 55
  Carmen Barba, Renzo Guerrini

- Differential diagnosis between epilepsy and particular forms of migraine with prolonged neurological symptoms in children. 71
  Dominique Parain

- Epilepsy and familial hemiplegic migraine. Genetic and clinical aspects 99
  Axel Lebas, Évelyne Guégan-Massardier, Lucie Guyant-Maréchal

- Treatments: overlap between migraine and epilepsy in children... 109
  Jean-Christophe Cuvellier, Louis Vallée

Comorbidity of epilepsy and migraine: epidemiological considerations

Dale C. Hesdorffer
New York, USA

Comorbidity is defined as the co-occurrence of two supposedly separate disorders at above chance levels (Rutter, 1994). There are several potential explanations for observed comorbidity of two disorders. It is possible that disorder A causes disorder B or *vice versa*. Another possibility is that disorder A and disorder B co-occur due to a common risk factor. If such a risk factor exists, then an intervention that is designed to reduce the occurrence of both disorders will only have an effect if it targets the common underlying risk factor. Shared genetic factors would operate in a similar manner to shared environmental risk factors. Disorder A and disorder B may be comorbid if they share an underlying characteristic that is part of the diagnosis of both conditions. Study methodology and bias may also lead to the observation that disorders A and B are comorbid. This may arise due to differences in the threshold for endorsing symptoms and behaviors. It is well-known that hospital-based studies of comorbidity can be biased. For example, Berkson's bias is a mathematical phenomenon that stipulates that the likelihood of hospitalization for one disorder is greater when a second disorder is also present than for either disorder alone. Clinical selection bias, which can also account for comorbidity, is the ascertainment of cases with the comorbid disorder under study to an extent greater than present in the community, because, for example, there is an increased probability of seeking care for disorder A when disorder B is also present. This chapter reviews the epidemiology of the comorbidity of migraine and epilepsy and briefly addresses several potential underlying mechanisms that might explain the co-occurrence of these disorders.

Definitions, prevalence and incidence

Epilepsy and migraine are both episodic disorders and they share some overlapping symptoms *(Table I)*, particularly for partial seizures. In some cases, seizures can follow a migraine aura (migralepsy), though this was found in only 3% of epilepsy in one large series (Velioglu *et al.*, 2005) and in 16% of patients with both epilepsy and migraine in another series (Marks and Ehrenberg, 1993). Migralepsy is, therefore, an unlikely explanation for the comorbidity of these disorders.

Table I. Aura in migraine and epilepsy

Symptom	Migraine	Epilepsy
Duration of aura	15-60 minutes	Brief, often < 1 minute
Automatisms	Unusual	Frequent for complex partial seizures
Gastrointestinal aura	Abdominal pain (rare) Nausea (common)	"Butterflies" – rising epigastric sensation
Visual disturbances	Positive/negative	Complex visual phenomenon
Paresthesias	Common (5-60 minutes)	Common (seconds to minutes)
Altered consciousness	Usually responsive	Often unresponsive
Olfactory	Very uncommon	More common
Aphasia	Uncommon	Common
Déjà vu	Rare	Common

Reproduced with permission from: Bigal ME, Lipton RB, Cohen J, Silberstein SD. Epilepsy and migraine. *Epilepsy and Behavior* 2003: 4: s13-S24.

Although epilepsy and migraine share some similar symptoms and migraine aura can directly precede a seizure, the prevalence and incidence of the two disorders differ. As can be seen below, epilepsy is considerably rarer than migraine, females predominate for migraine, except in children, whereas the reverse is true for epilepsy, and the age at peak occurrence differs.

Epilepsy

Epilepsy is defined as recurrent unprovoked seizures and as the occurrence of two or more unprovoked seizures for epidemiological studies (Commission on Epidemiology and Prognosis, 1993).

The prevalence of epilepsy shows wide variation across studies, but generally ranges from 4 to 10 per 1,000 population (Hauser *et al.*, 1991; Cowan *et al.*, 1989; Placencia *et al.*, 1994). This two- to three-fold variation is related in part to varying definitions, but it is also related to true differences in frequency across populations. The prevalence of epilepsy generally is higher in developing countries than in industrialized nations. In industrialized countries, prevalence tends to increase with advancing age, reaching a peak in the oldest age groups. In contrast, prevalence in developing countries is highest in young adults. Prevalent cases are highly selected from the population with incident epilepsy, because prevalent cases are characterized by chronicity and by survival from diagnosis. When prevalent cases are ascertained from the general population, they generally have much less severe disease than prevalent cases ascertained only through tertiary referral centers. This difference in severity must be taken into account when considering studies of the comorbidity of migraine and epilepsy from tertiary referral centers.

Studies of the incidence of epilepsy identify people with a new diagnosis of epilepsy in a defined population. Such a diagnosis is made after the patient sees a physician due to at least two unprovoked seizures. It is much easier to recognize two generalized tonic-clonic seizures than two absence or two complex partial seizures, and patients with these latter seizure types tend to be diagnosed later in the course of their epilepsy. Thus, the inception of incident cases of epilepsy is probably not homogeneous, but depends upon characteristics of the seizures. Incident cohorts are, therefore, heterogeneous for the number of seizures preceding diagnosis and the duration of epilepsy prior to diagnosis.

There are only a few total population incidence studies of epilepsy. The incidence of epilepsy in industrialized countries is about 50 per 100,000 population per year (Ólafsson et al., 2005; Hauser et al., 1993). The incidence in developing countries is probably double this rate (Placencia et al., 1994; Lavados et al., 1992). Regardless of geographic area, there is an excess incidence in males, and only about 35% of cases have a clearly identified antecedent. In industrialized countries, incidence is high in children up to 1 year, levels off by age 20, remains constant until age 60 and then climbs again in the elderly. This contrasts with developing countries, where incidence generally peaks in childhood and few new-onset cases are identified in adults after the age of 50 years.

Migraine

Migraine is a chronic disorder characterized by a least 5 episodes of headache lasting 4 to 72 hours with a number of associated characteristics (unilateral localization, pulsating quality, moderate to severe intensity, aggravation by routine physical activity) and associated symptoms (nausea and/or vomiting, photophobia and phonophobia) in the absence of another disorder that might explain the occurrence of such headaches (Headache Classification Committee of the International Headache Society, 2004). In the International Headache Society (IHS) definition (2004), migraine is further classified as migraine with aura (MA) and migraine without aura (MO). Some have suggested that MA and MO are different disease entities (Russell et al., 1996; Goadsby 2001), an assertion supported by familial aggregation and twin studies (Ulrich et al., 1999; Russell and Olesen, 1995). Additionally, a stronger genetic component has been found for MA than for MO (Russell and Olesen, 1995).

The lifetime prevalence of migraine was 14.7% in a health plan (Patel, 2004) with a female preponderance. The lifetime prevalence of MA was 7.9% in a Danish general population sample (Russell et al., 1996). Using the IHS definition, the one-year prevalence of migraine ranges from 3.0% to 10.6% (Mortimer et al., 1992; Abus-Arefeh et al., 1995; Raieli et al., 1995; Barea et al., 1996). Gender-specific prevalence is affected by age with a higher prevalence in boys than in girls before puberty and a reversal after puberty. Migraine prevalence peaks during adulthood and drops off beginning at about age 60 years.

There is less available information on the incidence of migraine. In a population-based study from Denmark (Lyngberg et al., 2005), the incidence of migraine meeting IHS criteria was assessed in a 12-year follow-up study of a general population (1989-2001) in which the prevalence of migraine was first assessed 12 years before the reassessment for migraine incidence. Among the 740 people (aged 25-64 years) evaluated in 1989, 673 were eligible in 2001 and 549 (81.6%) participated. The incidence of migraine was 8.1 per 1,000 person-years with a male: female ratio of 1:6. The incidence of migraine has also been estimated in a follow-up of an adult cohort aged 21-30 years from the general population. In this study, the incidence of migraine was 5.0 per 1,000 person-years for males and 22.0 for females, a 1: 4.4 ratio (Breslau et al., 1994).

While epilepsy and migraine share some symptoms and are both heterogeneous disorders, there are several interesting differences in their incidence and prevalence. The gender ratio differs for migraine *versus* epilepsy. For migraine, males predominate before puberty and females strongly predominate afterwards. In contrast, males predominate at all ages for epilepsy. The age at peak incidence also differs. The peak age for migraine (Lyngberg et al., 2005) is during the working years and for epilepsy (Ólafsson et al., 2005), it is under the age of one year and over the age of 60 years *(Fig. 1)*.

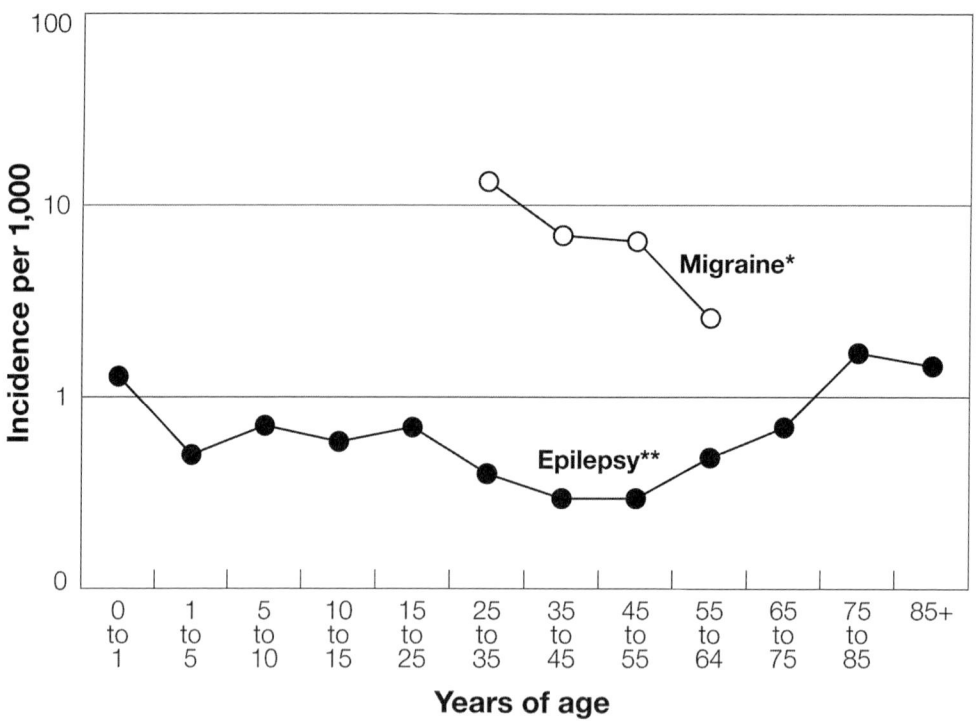

* Lyngberg AC, et al. Am J Epidemiol 2005; 161: 1066-73.

** Ólafsson E, et al. Lancet Neurology 2005; 4: 627-34.

Figure 1. Incidence of epilepsy and migraine.

Associations between migraine and epilepsy

Several studies have shown that migraine and epilepsy are comorbid, although time order is only assessed in two studies (Ottman and Lipton, 1994; Ludvigsson et al., 2006). Published studies have been based upon volunteers from an epilepsy advocacy organization, clinical series from a neurology department of tertiary centers that specialize in the diagnosis and treatment of epilepsy, and one population-based case-control study. When cases with epilepsy are drawn from voluntary organizations or from tertiary care centers, the cases are more likely to be severe with respect to seizure frequency, duration of epilepsy, and resistance to antiepileptic drug therapy. Thus, it can be seen that the selection of cases based on a characteristic of the epilepsy (*e.g.*, severity), which may lead people to seek care at a specialty clinic, might affect the results of the study if the characteristic is related to the co-occurrence of migraine. As has long been known, population-based studies remain the cleanest way to avoid any selection bias that could be present in the other series.

Leniger *et al.* (2003) conducted a study in outpatient clinics for epilepsy and migraine to determine whether clinical characteristics differed in 61 patients with both epilepsy and migraine compared to 280 patients with only epilepsy and 248 patients with only migraine. A standardized questionnaire was used to assess hemicrania, pulsating quality, moderate to severe pain intensity, worsening on physical activity, and associated symptoms (vomiting, nausea, sensibility for noise and light). Compared to patients with only migraine, patients with epilepsy and migraine were more likely to have aura (25.8% *vs.* 41.0%, p = 0.02), moderate to severe headache intensity (42.7% *vs.* 77.1%, $p < 0.001$), headache worsening on activity (56.5% *vs.* 78.7%, p = 0.001), phonophobia (56.5% *vs.* 80.3%, p = 0.001), and photophobia (54.4% *vs.* 78.7%, p = 0.001). When patients with migraine and epilepsy were compared to patients with epilepsy only, there was no difference in seizure type or epilepsy syndrome. The proportion of females was significantly higher in patients with comorbid epilepsy and migraine and patients with migraine only compared to patients with epilepsy only (80.3% and 83.1% *vs.* 49.3%, p = 0.001); age did not differ by group. This gender difference may be real or it may reflect a potential tendency for women with both epilepsy and migraine to seek care more often than women with only one of these conditions.

In a cross-sectional population-based study conducted from 1995-1998, using the UK General Practice Research Database, Gaitatzis *et al.* (2004) compared the prevalence of migraine in adults with epilepsy who were registered with primary care physicians to that of a similar group of adults without epilepsy. Migraine was defined by the presence of an ICD-9 diagnosis of 346 in the medical record. Overall, migraine was 1.6-fold more common in epilepsy (95%, CI = 1.4-1.8). Further exploration showed that this association was limited to individuals age 16-64 years, where migraine was 1.6-fold more likely to occur in people with epilepsy than in those without (95% CI = 1.5-1.8). The association was observed for men (RR = 2.2; 95% CI = 1.8-2.7) and for women (RR = 1.4; 95% CI = 1.3-1.7), and was less pronounced among individuals aged 64 and older (overall RR = 1.2; 95% CI = 0.8-2.0). It is possible that to the extent that individuals with migraine do not seek care for their headaches (Lipton *et al.*, 1997), migraine may be underestimated in this study. Also, to the degree to which individuals with one diagnosis (*i.e.*, epilepsy) may be more likely to report another neurological diagnosis (*i.e.*, migraine), there may be an association between migraine and epilepsy due to a diagnostic bias rather than to the presence of a true association.

Ottman and Lipton (1994) assessed the comorbidity of epilepsy and migraine in a cohort of 1,948 adults probands with epilepsy, recruited form 10 epilepsy voluntary organizations, and from 1,441 of their parents and siblings. Probands and their parents and siblings were interviewed using semistructured interviews. Migraine was defined as two or more severe headaches with at least two of the following symptoms: unilateral pain, throbbing pain, visual aura, or nausea. Age of onset of migraine headaches was also assessed and used to calculate the cumulative incidence of migraine in people with epilepsy. There was an increased risk for migraine in probands and in relatives with epilepsy compared to relatives without epilepsy (RR = 2.4; 95% CI = 2.0-2.8 for probands and RR = 2.4; 95% CI = 1.6-3.8 for relatives with epilepsy). While the risk for migraine was increased for subgroups of probands described by age at epilepsy onset, seizure type, and family history of epilepsy, the magnitude of the increased risk did not differ across these groups. However, probands with seizures associated with prior head injury had an increased risk for migraine that exceeded that for probands with idiopathic/cryptogenic seizures (RR = 4.1; 95% CI = 2.9-5.7 for probands with head injury and RR = 2.3; 95% CI = 1.9-2.7 for idiopathic/cryptogenic seizures). Since the interviews involved a retrospective assessment of age of onset of epilepsy and of migraine, misclassification of the temporal relationship between these conditions may be present. Results may also be affected by the source of probands. To the extent that individuals who belong to voluntary organizations for people with epilepsy are different from all individuals with prevalent epilepsy, one difference may be the tendency to have more than one neurological condition, in this case migraine. This could lead to an overestimation of the relationship between epilepsy and migraine. However, if there was an overestimation in this study it was likely to be relatively minor, because the association was also found in affected relatives of probands.

A study by Ludviggson *et al.* (2006) evaluated whether a history of migraine is associated with an increased risk for developing unprovoked seizures in children. The investigators established a nationwide surveillance system in Iceland to identify all children aged 5 through 15 years with newly diagnosed epilepsy or first unprovoked seizure (N = 145) from December 1995 through February 1999. For each case, two controls (N = 317) were selected as the next same sex births who were not a sibling of the case, were alive, resided in Iceland at the time of the index seizure, and did not have a history of unprovoked seizure on the date of the case's incident seizure were selected from the population registry as controls. A structured interview was used to assess duration of headache, headache characteristics, associated symptoms and recurrence. This information was used to make a modified IHS diagnosis of migraine. The criteria used for migraine differed from the IHS criteria in two ways. First, children with recurrent (*i.e.*, at least 2) episodes of migrainous headache were considered to have migraine, rather than the more rigorous criteria of 5 or more episodes described in the IHS criteria. Second, visual symptoms (zigzag lines, heat waves, blurry vision or loss of vision) were the only symptom explored for MA. These symptoms are overwhelmingly the most common aura (Lee and Olness, 1997). Cases without these visual symptoms were classified as MO. The risk for developing unprovoked seizures was increased

3.7-fold by a history of migraine (95% CI: 1.6-8.3). The association was stronger for females than males, for partial than generalized seizures, and for those with epilepsy than those with single unprovoked seizures. Migraine history was associated with a 4.1-fold increased risk for epilepsy (95% CI = 1.4-12.0) and a 3.2-fold increased risk for first unprovoked seizure (95% CI = 0.9-11.0). There was no increase in risk for unprovoked seizures in children with MO (OR = 1.4, 95% CI = 0.5-4.0); however, risk for unprovoked seizures was increased in children with MA (OR = 8.2; 95% CI = 2.3-28.9). The increased risk for children with MA was seen across seizure types and etiologies. Associations between MA and epilepsy were also found in a study of Finnish families with migraine but were limited to males (Artto *et al.*, 2006).

Studies have examined the prevalence of migraine in Benign Rolandic Epilepsy (BRE) (Giroud *et al.*, 1989; Wirrell and Hamiwka, 2006; Ludvigsson *et al.*, 2006), but only one has examined time order (Ludvigsson *et al.*, 2006). Wirrell and Hamiwka (2006) conducted a cross sectional study to assess whether migraine was more common in 53 children with BRE compared with 53 children with cryptogenic or symptomatic partial epilepsy and with 53 healthy controls. They found that definite or probable migraine were equally common in children with BRE as in those with cryptogenic/symptomatic epilepsy (11.3% in both), but children in both groups were more likely to have migraine than healthy controls (11.3% *vs.* 1.9%, p = 0.05). Similarly, in the Iceland study, migraine was associated with the greatest increased risk for BRE, but the association between migraine and epilepsy was universal, and not limited to a specific syndrome, seizure subtype, or cause.

In summary, studies have shown that the co-occurrence of migraine and epilepsy is more common in females (Ottman and Lipton, 1994; Leniger *et al.*, 2003). Patients with MA are 1.6 times more likely to have epilepsy than those with only migraine (p = 0.02; Leniger *et al.*, 2003). The association between epilepsy and migraine is bidirectional. The risk for new-onset migraine is increased in people with a history of epilepsy (Ottman and Lipton, 1994) and the risk for a first unprovoked seizure is increased 3.7-fold (95% CI = 1.6-8.3) in children with a history of migraine, due to MA (OR = 8.2; 95% CI = 2.3-28.9)(Ludvigsson *et al.*, 2006). While migraine is associated with BRE, this association is similar to that seen for other syndromes, seizure types and causes. Migraine may also be associated with childhood epilepsy with occipital paroxysms (Andermann and Zifkin, 1998).

Does comorbid migraine affect the prognosis of epilepsy?

A study has shown that the prognosis of epilepsy is worse in the presence of migraine (Velioglu *et al.*, 2005). This study evaluated the effect of a past history of migraine on the prognosis of prevalent epilepsy in 59 patients with epilepsy and migraine and 56 patients with epilepsy only who were followed for 5 to 10 years. The group with epilepsy and migraine was less likely to be seizure-free over 10 years compared with the group with epilepsy only (about 5% seizure-free in the epilepsy and migraine group at 6 years compared to about 25% in the epilepsy only group, p < 0.0001). Additionally, compared to the epilepsy only group, the epilepsy and migraine group had a longer duration of epilepsy, a lower early treatment response, and a higher incidence of intractable epilepsy and achieving remission with polytherapy, and more seizure control and medication problems for at least the last 2 years of follow-up. While this study is the first to suggest that comorbid migraine is associated with poorer outcome of epilepsy, it is limited by a small sample size and the choice of a prevalent rather than an incident cohort.

The role of major depression and suicide attempt in the comorbidity of migraine and epilepsy

Major depression and suicide attempt are comorbid with both migraine and with epilepsy *(Fig. 2)*. These overlapping relationships may further hone our understanding of the phenotype that gives rise to the epilepsy-migraine comorbidity. This section provides a review of the studies that have examined comorbidity of epilepsy with depression and suicide attempt and comorbidity of migraine with depression and suicide attempt.

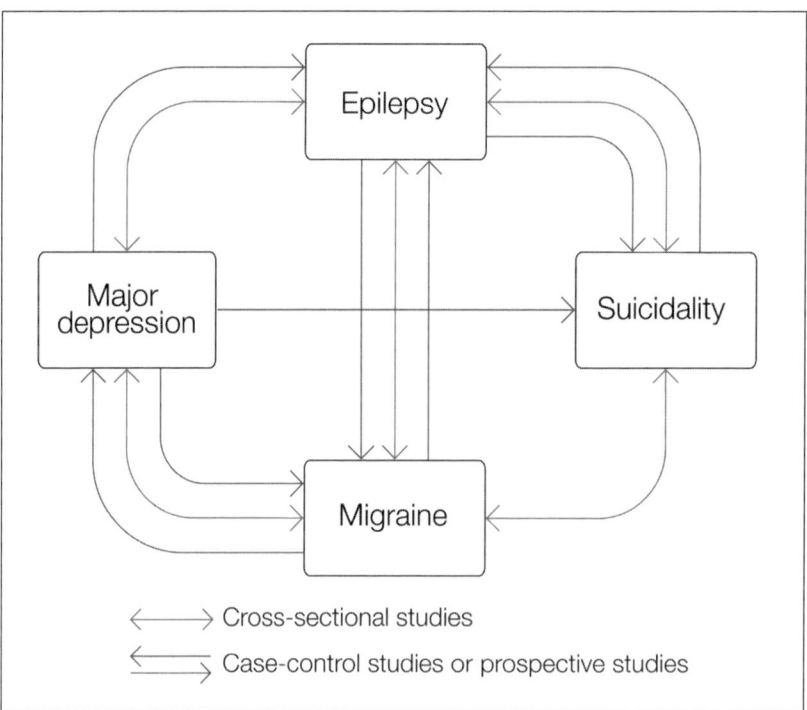

Reproduced with permission from: Hesdorffer DC. Comorbidity of epilepsy and neuropsychiatric disorders: epidemiological considerations. *In*: Ryvlin P, Beghi E, Camfield P, Hesdorffer D, eds. *From First Unprovoked Seizure to Newly Diagnosed Epilepsy*. Paris: John Libbey Eurotext, 2007, 71-95.

Figure 2. Relationships between epilepsy, migraine, major depression, and suicidality.

Epilepsy, depression and suicide attempt

Several studies indicate that major depression is comorbid with epilepsy, but methodological problems exist. Most studies have been cross-sectional (see for example, Cramer *et al.*, 2004; O'Donoghue *et al.*, 1999; Boylan *et al.*, 2004; Jacoby *et al.*, 1996; Dominian *et al.*, 1963; Beghi *et al.*, 2002) and find that depression occurs more often than expected among people with epilepsy. Others are conducted in select populations from epilepsy centers with resulting over-representation of complex partial seizures refractory to medication. None of the studies use instruments from which DSM diagnoses of depression can be made. In these cross-sectional studies, a moderate to severe number of symptoms of depression occurs in approximately 20% of people with prevalent epilepsy. In community surveys, 10%-24% of people with epilepsy have a moderate or severe number of depressive symptoms (Cramer *et al.*, 2004; O'Donoghue *et al.*, 1999). In contrast, 29.7% of people with an epilepsy in a monitoring unit (Boylan *et al.*, 2004) report depression, reflecting either selection factors or real differences by seizure severity. Real differences by seizure severity is the more likely explanation as two community surveys of patients with prevalent epilepsy from the British general practice system showed a positive correlation between seizure frequency and prevalence of depressive symptoms (Jacoby *et al.*, 1996, O'Donoghue *et al.*, 1999). In these studies, a moderate to severe number of depressive symptoms occurred in 4%-20% of cases in remission, 10%-39% in those with less than one seizure per month, and 21%-55% of those with one or more seizures per month. These studies suggest that either depression is a reaction to having seizures due to the uncertain timing of seizures and associated stigma; or the pathology that leads to frequent seizures in epilepsy is also associated with depression.

Based upon cross-sectional studies, many clinical epileptologists believe that the co-occurrence of depression and epilepsy is limited to individuals with epilepsy involving the limbic system. This impression may have originated with biased samples from studies restricted to patients at specialized epilepsy centers, which contain an excess of patients with complex partial seizures, because they are more likely to be intractable than other types of epilepsy. However, one cross-sectional study (Beghi *et al.*, 2002) based at a tertiary referral center, minimized selection bias associated with referral of the most severe epilepsy case to tertiary centers, by restricting the analysis to patients with prevalent idiopathic/cryptogenic epilepsy who were initially diagnosed at that center. In that study, 60% of patients had generalized seizures and 63% were without seizures for 12 months or more, suggesting that this is a less severe population with epilepsy than the total population seen at tertiary referral centers. Compared with blood donors, people with epilepsy were 11.3-fold (95% CI = 1.4-247.8) more likely to have moderate to severe depression with no difference by seizure type. Thus, associations between prevalent epilepsy and depression are not confined to prevalent complex partial seizures or to individuals with the most frequent seizures.

Studies suggest that a history of major depression is associated with an increased risk for *developing* unprovoked seizures, suggesting a common underlying susceptibility. Dominian *et al.* (1963) originally suggested that depression might precede epilepsy and observed that 16% of 51 patients with late-onset prevalent epilepsy had a history of depression before the initial seizure.

In a hospital-based retrospective cohort study, Nilsson *et al.* (2003) found an increased risk for developing epilepsy over a 10-year period in 13,748 patients hospitalized for major depression or bipolar disorder compared to 81,380 controls hospitalized for osteoarthritis and 69,149 controls hospitalized for diabetes. These authors found that adjustment for alcohol or drug "abuse" diminished the magnitude of the increased risk for epilepsy in individuals hospitalized for depression. Generalizability of these findings is limited by the use of hospitalized depression, because fewer than half of people who meet criteria for major depression seek medical care, and even fewer are hospitalized (Olfson et al., 2005; Kessler et al., 1999). Clinical selection bias could also account for the impact of substance abuse on the association between epilepsy and major depression in this study.

Population-based case-control studies also consistently demonstrate that a history of depression is associated with an increased risk for developing an isolated unprovoked seizure or newly diagnosed epilepsy. In the first of these studies conducted by Forsgren and Nystrom (1990), a history of depression was associated with a 7-fold increased risk of developing unprovoked seizure ($p = 0.03$) in Swedish adults. When analyses were restricted to cases with a "localized onset" seizure, depression was 17 times more common among cases than among controls ($p = 0.002$). Because patients responded to the questionnaire 4 to 6 weeks after the diagnosis of their first seizure, it is possible that responses were not limited to depression preceding the first diagnosis of epilepsy.

Two other studies have found that a history of depression, diagnosed according to DSM criteria, increased the risk of developing unprovoked seizure. Among older adults residing in Rochester, Minnesota (Hesdorffer et al., 2000), a history of major depression was associated with a 6-fold increased risk of developing a first idiopathic/cryptogenic unprovoked seizure (95% CI = 1.56-22). After adjusting for medical therapies for depression, including electroconvulsive shock therapy, antidepressants, and antipsychotics, major depression was 3.7 fold more common (95% CI = 0.8-17) before the case's seizure came to medical attention than among controls. This increased risk was most prominent among cases with partial-onset seizures. Among cases, major depression occurred closer to the index date than for controls, suggesting that pathophysiology leading to depression may lower seizure threshold in older adults.

In an Icelandic population-based case-control study (Hesdorffer et al., 2006) of 324 children and adults aged 10 years and older with first unprovoked seizure or newly diagnosed epilepsy and 647 age and gender matched controls, a history of major depression diagnosed according to DSM-IV criteria was associated with a 1.7-fold increased risk for developing epilepsy (95% CI = 1.1-2.7). This increased risk was also present in the subgroup with idiopathic/cryptogenic seizures (OR = 1.9, 95% CI = 1.1-3.3), even after adjustment for cumulative alcohol consumption.

Significant strengths of these population-based case-control studies are that: they were limited to incident unprovoked seizure and incident epilepsy, and are therefore able to address the time order of the association by examining a history of major depression before the first unprovoked seizure; controls were drawn from the population; major depression was diagnosed according to DSM criteria, using standardized instruments; and the association was evaluated separately in the subgroup with idiopathic/cryptogenic unprovoked seizure, thus eliminating causes of seizures (e.g., stroke, head injury) that are themselves associated with depression. Adjustment for alcohol consumption in the Icelandic study did not alter the association between major depression and epilepsy, ruling out one possible shared environmental risk factor.

One study has suggested that associations between depression and epilepsy may be caused by disturbances in neurotransmitter function common to depression, suicide attempt and seizures. In a recent cohort study, examining seizures as adverse events in FDA randomized clinical trials of SSRIs and SNRIs conducted between 1985 and 2000 (Alper et al., 2007), the risk for seizures in the placebo group with major depression was 19-fold that expected in the general population.

The association between suicide and epilepsy was first described by Pudhomme (1941). Originally, it was thought that people with epilepsy became suicidal due to their seizure disorder. This belief was later supported by studies showing that completed suicide occurs more often than expected in people with epilepsy than in the general population (Jones et al., 2003; Nilsson et al., 1997; Rafnsson et al., 2001; Barraclough 1987; Henriksen et al., 1970). Standardized mortality ratios for suicide in people with epilepsy range from 3.5 (Nilsson et al., 1997) to 5.0 (Rafnsson et al., 2001), and the proportionate mortality ratio ranges from 0.7% (Barraclough 1987) to 20% (Henriksen et al., 1970) when studies with at least 100 deaths are examined. Although the long held explanation for this finding was that depression leads to suicide in people with epilepsy, in part because their epilepsy makes them severely depressed, recent findings suggest that this explanation is unlikely. Rather it appears that suicidality can precede the development of a first unprovoked seizure. In the Icelandic population-based study (Hesdorffer et al., 2006), suicide attempt was associated with a 3.5-fold increased risk for *developing* epilepsy (95% CI = 1.5-8.6), after adjusting for major depression, bipolar disorder, and cumulative alcohol intake. Thus, parallel to the results of studies concerning major depression and epilepsy, suicidal behaviors *precede* the occurrence of a first unprovoked seizure. In a parallel study assessing the risk for suicide in people with epilepsy and controlling for a history of depression, Christensen et al. (2007) found that compared with controls, epilepsy was associated with an increased risk for completed suicide without regard for a history of psychiatric illness. Because others have shown that suicide attempt increases the risk of later completed suicide (Suominen et al., 2004), the increased risk for completed suicide in people with epilepsy may reflect the recurrence of premorbid suicidal behavior rather than epilepsy leading to major depression and completed suicide. These results further suggest a common underlying susceptibility to epilepsy and suicidal behavior that is independent of major depression and bipolar disorder.

Migraine, depression and suicide attempt

Analogous to studies of epilepsy *(Fig. 2)*, migraine is also associated with both major depression and with suicide attempt (Breslau et al., 1991; Breslau and Davis, 1993; Breslau et al., 2000; Fasmer and Oedegaard, 2001; Lipton et al., 2000). The association between major depression and migraine is bidirectional and is strongest for MA (Breslau et al., 2000). Suicide attempt is also more common in migraine compared to controls, and the association is strongest for MA, even after adjusting for depression (Breslau et al., 1991).

Several studies (Breslau et al., 1991; Breslau and Davis 1993; Breslau et al., 2003) have evaluated the association between major depression, suicide attempt and migraine. These studies contribute to our understanding of the cross-sectional associations as well as the risk for migraine among people with major depression and the risk for major depression among people with migraine.

A cross-sectional study conducted in a random sample of 1,200 adults, aged 21-30 years, from a health maintenance organization in Detroit (Breslau et al., 1991) examined the prevalence of migraine in prevalent depression. Major depression was 2.2-fold more common in migraine without aura *versus* controls (95% CI = 1.2-4.0) and was 4.0-fold more common in migraine with aura than in controls (95% CI = 2.2-7.2). Suicide attempt was not associated with migraine without aura, but was 3.0-fold more common in migraine with aura than in controls (95% CI = 1.4-6.6). In a 14-month follow-up of the same cohort (Breslau and Davis, 1993), new psychiatric disorders over the follow-up period were ascertained for 99.1% of the cohort. Compared to those without a history of migraine, people with a history of migraine were 9.5-fold more likely to develop panic disorder with depression (95% CI = 1.3-69.6), 2.5-fold more likely to develop depression without panic (95% CI = 1.0-6.5) and 25.2-fold more likely to develop panic and depression (95% CI = 2.5-250.9). Thus, associations between major depression and suicide attempt are stronger for migraine with aura than for migraine without aura, although these differences do not reach statistical significance.

Three studies (Breslau et al., 2003; Swartz et al., 2000; Lipton et al., 2000) have evaluated the temporal nature of associations between migraine and major depression. The first (Swartz et al., 2000) was a nested case-control study in the Baltimore Epidemiological Catchment Area Study. Cases were incident migraine identified between the baseline interview in 1981 and the follow-up interviews in 1993 and 1996. Controls were individuals who did not report migraine at any interview. Major depression was not associated with incident migraine; however, in cross-sectional analysis, prevalent major depression was associated with prevalent migraine (OR = 2.2; 95% CI = 1.4-3.5 after adjustment for age and gender). The second study (Breslau et al., 2003) reported a bidirectional relationship between major depression and migraine. In this study, a representative sample of Detroit adults was evaluated in 1997 and again in 1999. 496 people with migraine were included in the study, 151 people with headache of comparable severity and 496 controls. Among controls, the presence of major depression in 1997 was associated with a 3.4-fold increased risk for new onset migraine in 1999 (95% CI = 1.4-8.7); there was no association between depression and other severe headaches. Migraine at baseline was associated with a 5.8-fold increased risk for major depression in 1999 (95% CI = 2.7-12.3), but again not for other severe headaches. There was no relationship between comorbid major depression and severity of migraine. In the third study (Lipton et al., 2000), two population-based studies of similar design conducted in the United States and in the United Kingdom were collapsed. At baseline, a telephone interview identified people with and without migraine and depression was assessed at follow-up. Depression occurred in 47% of 389 people with migraine compared with 17% of 379 people without migraine (adjusted prevalence ratio = 2.7; 95% CI = 2.1-3.5). Thus, two studies find that migraine increases the risk for depression (Breslau et al., 2003; Lipton et al., 2000) and one study finds that depression increases the risk for incident migraine (Breslau et al., 2003).

In considering whether the type of affective disorder may differ, according to the presence or absence of comorbid migraine, Fasmer and Oedegaard (2001) studied 102 patients with an index episode of major depression or mania (49 with migraine and 53 without migraine) who were admitted to a psychiatric ward, outpatient service or day-care unit of one hospital. Migraine was defined according to HIS criteria. There was no difference in the occurrence of unipolar depression, but bipolar I was more common in patient with comorbid migraine (23% *versus* 5%, p < 0.001) and bipolar II was less common in patients with comorbid migraine (6% *versus* 16%, p = 0.009). When features of major depressive episodes were compared in patients with and without comorbid migraine, only irritability (40% *versus* 26%, p = 0.02) and suspiciousness (39% *versus* 25%, p = 0.02) were significantly different in those with and without migraine. In contrast to other studies, suicide attempt did not differ by presence or absence of migraine in this cohort with affective disorder. In analyses examining anxiety disorder, the authors found that panic disorder and agoraphobia were significantly more common in patients with migraine.

Epilepsy, migraine, depression, and suicide attempt

The overlapping relationships between migraine, major depression, suicidality and epilepsy *(Fig. 2)* suggest that either migraine is a confounder of the relationship between major depression, suicidality and epilepsy or that there is a differential effect of depression or suicidality in the presence compared to the absence of migraine. These issues were examined in the Icelandic study among 324 individuals aged 10 and older with newly diagnosed unprovoked seizures 647 age- and gender-matched controls (Hesdorffer *et al.*, 2007). In these analyses, migraine was not a confounder of the relationship between major depression, suicidality and epilepsy. Further analyses examined whether the co-occurrence of MA with either major depression or with suicide attempt increases the risk for developing unprovoked seizure more than these conditions alone. Major depression with MA increased the risk for unprovoked seizures more than either condition alone (major depression and MA, OR = 4.6; major depression only, OR = 1.4; MA only, OR = 2.5). The same was seen for suicide attempt with MA (suicide attempt and MA, OR = 7.9; suicide attempt only, OR = 4.7; MA only, OR = 2.4). The number of conditions showed a linear relationship to seizure risk (OR = 2.0 with any one condition, OR = 4.9 with any two conditions, and OR = 6.7 with all three conditions); this linear trend was statistically significant. In a similar analysis from a follow-up of the health maintenance organization cohort, Breslau and Davis (1993) compared the occurrence of suicide attempt by the presence or absence of migraine and major depression and found that suicide attempts were 3.0-fold more common in migraine without depression (95% CI = 1.2-8.0), 7.6-fold more common in major depression without migraine (95% CI = 3.4-16.8) and 16.2-fold more common in migraine with major depression (95% CI = 6.7-39.4). Together, these findings may reflect a new condition cluster defined by MA, major depression, suicide attempt and unprovoked seizures.

Does familial aggregation explain comorbid epilepsy and migraine?

When migraine and epilepsy are examined and the other comorbid conditions ignored, shared genetic factors are not the explanation for the comorbidity of migraine and epilepsy in the one study to examine this (Ottman and Lipton 1996). In this study, the risk for migraine was assessed in 1,423 first degree relatives of 1957 adult probands with epilepsy. The authors hypothesized that if genetic factors explain the comorbidity, then the risk of migraine should be higher in relatives of probands with genetic forms of epilepsy than in relatives of probands with nongenetic forms (symptomatic epilepsies). Genetic etiology of the proband's epilepsy was not associated with migraine in relatives, indicating an absence of familial co-aggregation. The occurrence of migraine in relatives was also not associated with a family history of epilepsy, reinforcing the lack of familial co-aggregation. The proband's history of migraine was associated with migraine in the relatives (adjusted RR = 1.5; 95%CI = 1.2-2.1), confirming that migraine is familial. In analyses restricted to relatives, the risk for migraine was increased 2.3-fold when the relative also had a positive history of epilepsy (95% CI = 1.5-3.6), confirming prior studies of the comorbidity of migraine and epilepsy. Two possible methodological factors may explain the absence of familial co-aggregation of epilepsy and migraine in this study. First, the control group consisted of families of people with symptomatic seizures. To the extent that genetic factors linking susceptibility to migraine and to seizures exist regardless of seizure etiology, this control group would sharply attenuate a finding of familial co-aggregation. Second, shared genetic factors were studied in a select population of people with prevalent epilepsy who participate in voluntary organizations and are more likely to represent people with refractory partial seizures than a general population sample of people with prevalent epilepsy. If migraine and epilepsy are more likely to occur together in families with generalized forms of epilepsy, then this study was unlikely to detect the familial aggregation of these disorders.

Does familial aggregation explain the comorbidity of migraine and depression?

This topic is of interest because it is possible that shared genetic factors for epilepsy and migraine may be limited to the subgroup with migraine and depression. One study has examined the familial co-aggregation of major depression and migraine (Merikangas *et al.*, 1988). This study examined 400 adult first degree relatives of 133 probands with major depression and of 82 controls with no history of psychiatric illness or treatment either by history or by interview. Lifetime history of self-reported migraine was obtained by direct interview, but systematic data were not collected. This study confirmed that depression occurs in families and migraine occurs in families. It also confirmed that in individuals the two disorders are comorbid. However, results did not support a shared genetic susceptibility to migraine and depression in families. Among the 108 depressed probands without migraine, 6.7% of relatives had migraine compared with 8.6% of relatives of 76 control probands without migraine. A major limitation of this study is the method used to identify migraine. To the extent that a self-report of migraine results in misclassification, the results may be attenuated towards no effect.

Other possible explanations for the comorbidity of epilepsy and migraine

Migraine may lead to silent infarcts and to clinically-detected ischemic stroke, mechanisms that might explain both the increased risk for developing epilepsy in people with a history of migraine and the poor prognosis of epilepsy in the presence of a history of migraine. In a population-based cross-sectional study, Kruit *et al.* (2004) evaluated the presence of brain infarcts and white matter lesions in Dutch adults, aged 30 to 60 years. Included were a randomly selected subset of 161 adults with migraine with aura, 134 subjects with migraine without aura, and 161 controls who underwent an MRI examination. No subjects had prior transient ischemic attack or an abnormal neurological examination. While there were no differences between groups in the overall prevalence of infarction, there were differences with regard to the location of infarcts. Specifically, infarcts in the cerebellar region of the posterior circulation were 7.1-fold more common in migraine than in controls (95% CI = 0.9-55) and 13.7-fold more common in migraine with aura compared to controls (95% CI = 1.7-112). Increased frequency of migraine attacks was also associated with infarcts in this region (OR = 9.3; 95% CI = 1.1-76). A gender-specific effect was seen for the association between a high load of deep white matter lesions and migraine with an effect in women (OR = 2.1; 95%CI = 1.0-4.1) but not in men. There was no association between periventricular white matter lesions and migraine. While there have been no studies of subclinical lesions and risk for developing epilepsy, these data suggest that this question should be explored as a potential mechanism for the comorbidity of epilepsy and migraine and for the poor prognosis of epilepsy in association with a history of migraine. In two parallel analyses, one conducted in the Women's Health Study (Kurth *et al.*, 2006a) and the other in the Physician's Health Study (Kurth *et al.*, 2006b), Kurth *et al.* (2006a, 2006b) found that migraine was associated with an increased risk for clinically detected ischemic stroke in women, where the association was limited to migraine with aura (RR = 2.1, 95% CI = 1.3-3.3), but there was no association in men. This study suggests that some of the association between migraine and epilepsy in older adults may be mediated through ischemic stroke in women.

Channelopathies have been proposed as the underlying mechanism for several episodic disorders, including epilepsy and migraine (Terwindt *et al.*, 1998). Avanzini *et al.* (2007) have reviewed the evidence that some genetic epilepsies are associated with mutations in genes coding for subunits of voltage or ion-gated ligands and Barbas and Schuyler (2006) have done the same for migraine. To date, three genes have been identified in familial hemiplegic migraine: *ATP1A2*, *SCN1A* and *CACNA1A*. Of these, *SCN1A* has also been implicated in severe myoclonic epilepsy and in generalized epilepsy with febrile seizures plus.

Considerable evidence supports the comorbidity of convulsive disorders with migraine, particularly MA, and both of these disorders with major depression and suicide attempt. Most of the studies of epilepsy and migraine conducted to date cannot establish time order, but those that do find MA is associated with an increased risk for *developing* epilepsy and epilepsy is associated with an increased risk for *developing* migraine. Cross-sectional studies, which are much more difficult to interpret, support the association of these two conditions. Further clarification of these associations is needed in order to further understand their underpinnings, including attempts to further characterize phenotypes, to understand the role of potential common underlying risk factors and to elucidate any shared pathogenesis and shared genetic susceptibility. Such studies should use standardized validated instruments designed to make HIS diagnoses of migraine, include adequate numbers of people with first unprovoked seizure or newly diagnosed epilepsy, and have appropriate controls in order to better characterize these relationships.

References

- Abus-Arefeh I, Russell G. Prevalence and clinical features of abdominal migraine compared with those of migraine headache. *Arch Dis Chil* 1995; 72: 413-7.

- Alper K, Schwartz KA, Kolts RL, Khan A. Seizure Incidence in Psychopharmacological Clinical Trials: An Analysis of Food and Drug Administration (FDA) Summary Basis of Approval Reports. *Biol Psychiatry* 2007, in press and on line.

- Andermann F, Zifkin B. The benign occipital epilepsies of childhood: An overview of the idiopathic syndromes and of the relationship to migraine. *Epilepsia* 1998: 39 (suppl. 4): S9-S23.

- Artto V, Wessman M, Nissiliä M, *et al.* Comorbidity in Finnish migraine families. *J Headache Pain* 2006; 7: 324-330.

- Avanzini G, Franceschetti S, Mantegazza M. Epileptogenic channelopathies: Experimental models of human pathologies. *Epilepsia* 2007; 48 (suppl. 2): 51-64.

- Bakken K, Landheim AS, Vaglum P. Primary and secondary substance misusers: do they differ in substance-induced and substance-independent mental disorders? *Alcohol & Alcoholism* 2003; 38(1):54-9.

- Barbas NR, Schuyler EA. Heredity, genes, and headache. *Seminars in Neurology* 2006; 26: 507-14.

- Barea LM, Tannhauser M, Rotta NT. An epidemiologic study of headache among children and adolecents of southern Brazil. *Cephalalgia* 1996; 16: 545-9.

- Barraclough BM. The suicide rate of epilepsy. *Acta Psychiatr Scand* 1987; 76: 339-45.

- Beghi E, Spagnoli P, Airoldi L, *et al.* Emotional and affective disturbances in patients with epilepsy. *Epilepsy Behav* 2002; 3: 255-61.

- Boylan LS, Flint LA, Labovitz DL, *et al.* Depression but not seizure frequency predicts quality of life in treatment-resistant epilepsy. *Neurology* 2004; 62: 617-23.

- Breslau N, Davis GC, Andreski P. Migraine, psychiatric disorders, and suicide attempts: an epidemiologic study of young adults. *Psychiatry Res* 1991; 37: 11-23.

- Breslau N, Davis GC. Migraine, physical health and psychiatric disorder: A prospective epidemiologic study in young adults. *J Psychiat Res* 1993; 27: 211-21.

- Breslau N, Davis GC, Schultz LR, Peterson EL. Migraine and major depression. *Headache* 1994; 34: S17-S26.

- Breslau N, Schultz LR, Stewart WF, *et al.* Headache and major depression: is the association specific to migraine? *Neurology* 2000; 54: 308-13.

- Breslau N, Lipton RB, Stewart WF, *et al.* Comorbidity of migraine and depression: investigating potential etiology and prognosis. *Neurology* 2003; 60: 1308-12.

- Christensen J, Verseegaard M, Mortensen PB, *et al.* Epilepsy and risk of suicide: a population-based case-control study. *Lancet Neurology* 2007; 6: 693-8.

- Commission on Classification and Terminology of the International League Against Epilepsy. Guidelines for epidemiologic studies on epilepsy. *Epilepsia* 1993; 34: 592-6.

- Cowan LD, Leviton A, Bodensteiner JB, Doherty L. Problems in estimating the prevalence of epilepsy in children: the yield from different sources of information. *Paediatr Perinat Epidemiol* 1989; 3: 386-401.

- Cramer JA, Blum D. Fanning K, Reed M for the Epilepsy Impact Project. The impact of comorbid depression on health resource utilization in a community sample of people with epilepsy. *Epilepsy Behav* 2004; 337-42.

- Dominian MA, Serafetinides EA, Dewhurst M. A follow-up study of late-onset epilepsy: II. Psychiatric and social findings. *Br Med J* 1963; 1: 431-5.

- Fasmer OB, Oedegaard KJ. Clinical characteristics of patients with major affective disorders and comorbid migraine. *World J Biol Psychiatry* 2001; 2: 149-55.

- Forsgren L, Nystrom L. An incident case-referent study of epileptic seizures in adults. *Epilepsy Res* 1990; 6: 66-81.

- Gaitatzis A, Carroll K, Majeed A, Sander JW. The epidemiology of the comorbidity of epilepsy in the general population. *Epilepsia* 2004; 45: 1613-22.

- Giroud M, Couillault G, Arnould S, *et al*. Épilepsie à paroxysmes rolandiques et migraine, une association non fortuite. Résultats d'une étude contrôlée. *Pédiatrie* 1989; 44: 659-64.

- Goadsby PJ. Migraine, aura and cortical spreading depression: Why are we still talking about it? *Ann Neurol* 2001; 49: 4-5.

- Hauser WA, Annegers JF, Kurland LT. Prevalence of epilepsy in Rochester, Minnesota: 1940-1980. *Epilepsia* 1991; 32: 429-45.

- Hauser WA, Annegers JF, Kurland LT. Incidence of epilepsy and unprovoked seizures in Rochester, Minnesota: 1935-1984. *Epilepsia* 1993; 34: 453-68.

- Headache Classification Committee of the International Headache Society. Classification and diagnostic criteria for headache disorders, cranial neuroalgias, and facial pain. Second Edition. *Cephalalgia* 2004; suppl. 1: 1-160.

- Henriksen B, Juul-Jensen P, Lund M. Mortality of epileptics. In: Brackenridge R (ed). *Life Assurance Medicine*. London: Pitman, 1970, 139-48.

- Hesdorffer DC, Hauser WA, Annegers JF, Cascino G. Major depression is a risk factor for seizures in older adults. *Ann Neurol* 2000; 47: 246-9.

- Hesdorffer DC, Hauser WA, Ludvigsson P, *et al*. Depression and attempted suicide as risk factors for incident unprovoked seizures and epilepsy. *Ann Neurology* 2006; 59: 35-41.

- Hesdorffer DC, Ludvigsson P, Hauser WA, *et al*. Co-occurrence of major depression or suicide attempt and migraine with aura and risk factor for unprovoked seizure. *Epilepsy Research* 2007; 25: 220-3.

- Jacoby A, Baker GA, Stgeen N, *et al*. The clinical course of epilepsy and its psychosocial findings from a U.K. community study. *Epilepsia* 1996; 37: 148-61.

- Jones JE, Hermann BP, Bary JJ, *et al*. Rates and risk factors for suicide, suicidal ideation, and suicide attempts in chronic epilepsy. *Epilepsy Behav* 2003; 4: S31-S38.

- Kessler RC, Zhao S, Katz SJ, *et al*. Past-year use of outpatient services for psychiatric problems in the National Comorbidity Survey. *Am J Psychiatry* 1999; 156: 115-23.

- Kruit MC, van Buchem MA, Hofman PAM, *et al*. Migraine as a risk factor for subclinical brain lesions. *JAMA* 2004; 291: 427-34.

- Kurth T, Gaziano JM, Cook NR, *et al*. Migraine and risk of cardiovascular disease in women. *JAMA* 2006a; 296: 283-91.

- Kurth T, Gaziano JM, Cook NR, *et al*. Migraine and risk of cardiovascular disease in men. *Arch Intern Med* 2006b; 167: 795-801.

- Lavados J, Germain I, Morales A, *et al*. A descriptive study of epilepsy in the District of El Salvador, Chile 1984-1988. *Acta Neurol Scand* 1992; 91: 718-29.

- Leniger T, von den Driesch S, Isbruch K, *et al*. Clinical characteristics of patients with comorbidity of migraine and epilepsy. *Headache* 2003; 43: 672-7.

- Lipton RB, Stewart WF, von Korff M. Burden of migraine: societal costs and therapeutic opportunities. *Neurology* 1997; 48 (suppl. 3): S4-9.

- Lipton RB, Hamelsky SW, Kolodner KB, et al. Migraine, quality of life, and depression: a population-based case-control study. *Neurology* 2000; 55: 629-35.

- Ludvigsson P, Hesdorffer D, Olafsson E, et al. Migraine with aura is a risk factor for unprovoked seizures in children. *Ann Neurol* 2006; 59: 210-3.

- Lyngberg AC, Rasmussen BK, Jørgensen T, Jensen R. Incidence of primary headache: a Danish epidemiologic follow-up study. *Am J Epidemiol* 2005; 161: 1066-73.

- Marks DA, Ehrenberg BL. Migraine-related seizures in adults with epilepsy, with EEG correlation. *Neurology* 1993; 43: 2476-83.

- Merikangas KR, Risch NJ, Merikangas JR, et al. Migraine and depression: association and familial transmission. *J Psychiatr Res* 1988; 22: 119-29.

- Mortimer MJ, Kay J, Jaron A. Epidemiology of headache and childhood migraine in an urban general practice using Ad Hoc, Vahlquist and IHS criteria. *Dev Med Child Neurol* 1992; 34: 1095-101.

- Nilsson L, Tomson T, Farahmand BY, et al. Cause-specific mortality in epilepsy: A cohort study of more than 9,000 patients once hospitalized for epilepsy. *Epilepsia* 1997; 38: 1062-8.

- Nilsson FM, Kessing LV, Bolwig TG. On the increased risk of developing late-onset epilepsy for patients with major affective disorder. *J Affective Dis* 2003; 76: 39-48.

- O'Donoghue MF, Goodridge DM, Redhead K, et al. Assessing the psychosocial consequences of epilepsy: a community-based study. *Br J Gen Practice* 1999; 49: 211-4.

- Ólafsson E, Ludvigsson P, Gudmundsson G, et al. Incidence of unprovoked seizures and epilepsy: Limited usefulness of the epilepsy syndrome classification in a population-based study. *Lancet Neurology* 2005: 4: 627-34.

- Olfson M, Das AK, Gameroff MJ, et al. Bipolar depression in a low-income primary care clinic. *Am J Psychiatry* 2005; 162: 2146-51.

- Ottman R, Lipton RB. Comorbidity of migraine and epilepsy. *Neurology* 1994; 44: 2105.

- Ottman R, Lipton RB. Is the comorbidity of epilepsy and migraine due to a shared genetic susceptibility? *Neurology* 1996; 47: 918-24.

- Patel NV, Bigal ME, Kolodner KB, et al. Prevalence and impact of migraine and probable migraine in a health plan. *Neurology* 2004; 63: 1432-8.

- Placencia M, Sander JW, Roman M, et al. The characteristics of epilepsy in a largely untreated population in rural Ecuador. *J Neurol Neurosurg Psychiatry* 1994; 57: 320-50.

- Prudhomme C. Epilepsy and suicide. *J Nerv Ment Dis* 1941; 94: 722-31.

- Rafnsson V, Ólafsson E, Hauser WA. Cause-specific mortality in adults with unprovoked seizures: A population-based incidence cohort study. *Neuroepidemiology* 2001: 20: 232-6.

- Raieli V, Raimondo D. Gangitano M, et al. Migraine headaches in adolescents: a student population-based study in Monreale. *Cephalgia* 1995; 15: 5-12.

- Russel MB, Rasmussen BK, Fenger K, Olesen J. Migraine without aura and migraine with aura are distinct clinical entities: a study of four hundred and eighty-four male and female migraineurs from the general population. *Cephalagia* 1996; 16: 239-45.

- Rutter M. Comorbidity: Meanings and Mechanisms. *Clin Psychol Sci Prac* 1994; 1: 100-3.

- Suominen K, Isometsa E, Suokas J, et al. Completed suicide after suicide attempt: A 37-year follow-up study. *Am J Psychiatry* 2004; 161: 563-4.

- Swartz KL, Pratt LA, Armenian HK. Mental disorders and the incidence of migraine headaches in a community sample. *Arch Gen Psychiatry* 2000; 57: 945-0.

- Terwindt GM, Ophoff RA, Haan J, *et al.* for the Dutch Migraine Genetics Research Group. Migraine, ataxia and epilepsy: a challenging spectrum of genetically determined calcium channelopathies. *Eur J Human Genetics* 1998; 6: 297-307.

- Ulrich V, Gervil M, Kyvik KO, *et al.* The inheritance of migraine with aura estimated by means of structural equation modeling. *J Med Genet* 1999; 36: 225-7.

- Velioglu SK, Boz C, Özmenoglu M. The impact of migraine on epilepsy: a prospective prognosis study. *Cephalalgia* 2005; 25: 528-35.

- Wirrell EC, Hamiwka LD. Do children with Benign Rolandic Epilepsy have a higher prevalence of migraine than those with other partial epilepsies or nonepilepsy controls? *Epilepsia* 2006;47: 1674-81.

Migraine's pathophysiological mechanisms

Gilles Géraud
Toulouse, France

Migraine is a chronic disease characterized by recurring headache attacks. Most migraineurs present no symptoms between attacks, though some experience a more or less permanent hypersensitivity to light, noise or smell.

Migraine is a primary brain disease. Attacks originate somewhere in the brain by an inappropriate neuronal activation that triggers a cerebral vasomotor storm. Many possible triggering factors of an attack, plus numerous clinical signs associated with pain, have motivated for a long time and still motivate today searches for an extracerebral origin of the migraine (eyes, sinuses, teeth, neck, some foods, etc.). These strong beliefs drive some sufferers to seek help from many specialists, accumulating various paraclinical findings in a desperate search for an explanation that they are unlikely to find.

The mechanisms involved in the migraine are complex and still poorly understood. However, many significant advances have been made in the recent years and bit by bit the pieces of this puzzle are falling into place.

Origin of the attack

The source of the migraine attack in the brain is still unknown. Results from experimental research and clinical arguments suggest an origin within the hypothalamus and the superior part of the brainstem.

What we can learn from patients

Some migraineurs can predict the occurrence of an attack because of characteristic signs experienced a few hours and sometimes even a few days before. These so-called prodromes, are brought about by a temporary disturbance in homeostatic functioning controlling hunger, thirst, body temperature, awareness and mood. These functions are regulated by nuclei located in the hypothalamus and midbrain. It is thus tempting to localise the origin of the migraine attack to these areas of the brain.

Non migraineurs have been shown to develop headache syndromes resembling migraine attacks, following electrode implantation in the periaqueductal gray region (PAG) of the midbrain for the treatment of chronic pain (Raskin et al., 1987). New onset migraine has also been reported following bleeding of a cavernous angioma in the brain stem (Afridi and Goadsby, 2003).

Functional neuroimaging

It is only in 1995 that direct evidence for brain stem activation has been seen in migraineurs during spontaneous attacks. Using positron emission tomography (PET), Weiller *et al.* (1995) studied 9 patients, presenting with migraine without aura and right hemicrania, and observed a moderate increase in blood flow in the cingular, auditory and visual cortices. This increase in blood flow was abolished by sumatriptan suggesting a link with headache and phono- and photophobia. Increase in blood flow did however persist in the left posterior midbrain (close to the dorsal raphe nucleus and locus coeruleus) following sumatriptan-induced pain relief, suggesting a neuronal hyperactivity specific to the migraine process. These results have recently been confirmed and amplified by Denuelle *et al.* (2004) in 7 migraineurs who had been experiencing an attack for less than 6 hours. Activation of the hypothalamus, PAG, red nuclei, locus coeruleus contralateral to the pain and the posterior reticular formation were seen with a higher performance camera and computer program used to superimpose PET and magnetic resonance imaging (MRI) images. Following sumatriptan-induced pain relief, these activations persisted in the brain stem and hypothalamic region *(Fig. 1)*. Both studies strongly suggest an intense neuronal activation in the brain stem and hypothalamus

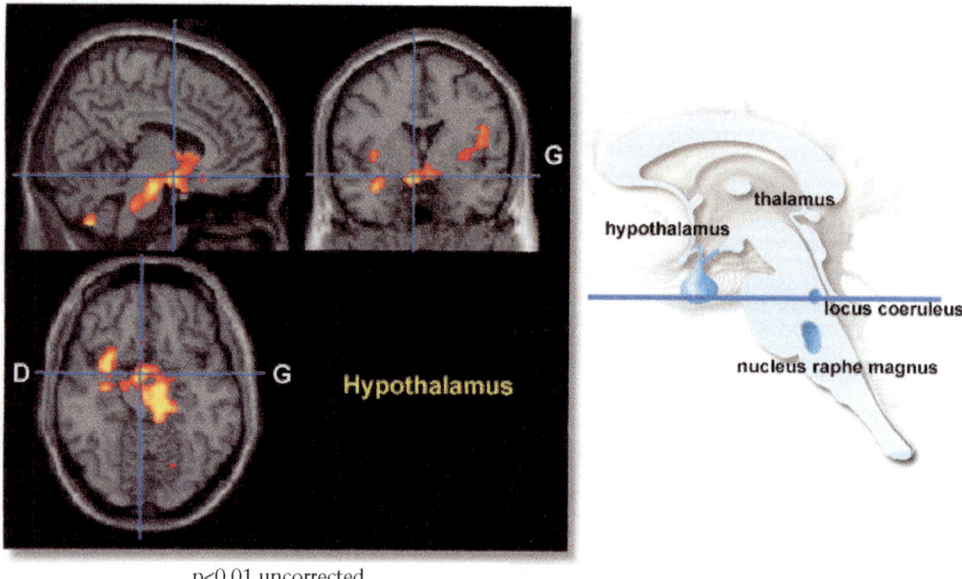

p<0.01 uncorrected

Figure 1. Activation at the the hypothalamus and brain stem level; recorded by PET during a spontaneous migraine attack without aura (7 patients). Recordings were carried out during the first 4 hours of attack (Denuelle *et al.*, 2007).

at the beginning of a migraine attack, which persists after treatment with triptan for the attack's symptoms. The persistence of this neuronal activation could explain the frequent recurrence of the headache after the effects of triptan have worn off. In the absence of sequential studies carried out at the period when attacks have just begun or even at the prodrome stage, it is impossible to be sure of the exact order of activation of these different structures and precisely where the process begins. However, clinical reasons outlined above lead us to predict that the origin of the migraine attack is located in the hypothalamic region.

Migraine aura

Fifteen to twenty percent of migraineurs present transitory visual symptoms before the headache, comprising a scintillating scotoma; *i.e.* a blind spot in the visual field, bordered by sparkling phosphenes forming a serated line. Purely specific to migraine scotoma, this effect starts off very small and close to the central visual field and spreads progressively within the peripheral visual field before complete hemifield invasion in 10 to 30 minutes.

Three dates, three authors

1941: Lashley studied his own visual migrainous scotoma and put it down to the architectonic organization of the visual cortex, estimating that it corresponds to a cortical excitation which spreads progressively along the striate cortex at a speed of 3 mm/min, followed by a period of inhibition *(Fig. 2)*.

Cortical spreading depression

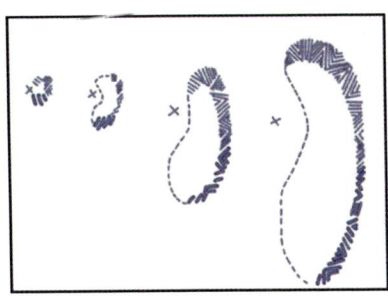

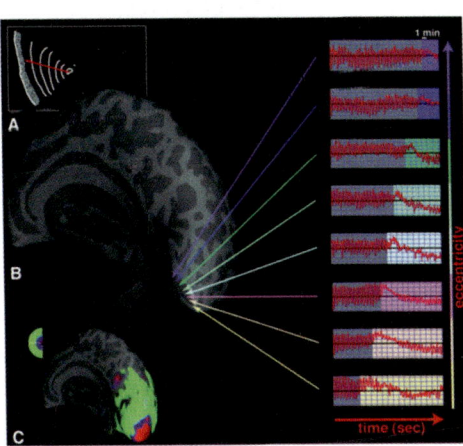

Original drawing by Lashley (1941)   Hadjikhani, PNAS 2001

Figure 2. Temporal evolution of the migraine visual scotoma (original drawing by Lashley) and functional MRI visualization of a CSD spreading along the occipital cortex at the back towards the front during a migraine with aura triggered following physical effort by an intermittent light stimulus (modified from Hadjikhani et al., 2001).

1944: The neurophysiologist Leao experimentally produced the same phenomena on the cortex of the rat and the cat, which he named cortical spreading depression (CSD).

1958: Milner hypothesized that the migrainous scotoma is a consequence of CSD, though this theory went more or less unnoticed in a time when interests were dominated by the works of Wolff and the vascular theory of migraine relating the aura to cortical ischemia caused by arterial spasm.

Cortical spreading depression

Cortical spreading depression (CSD) is a wave of neuronal and glial depolarization spreading from a site of initiation in all directions at a speed of 2 to 5 mm/min. Though very difficult to reproduce in the human brain, possibly due to cortical folding, the CSD has recently been reported when Hadjikhani *et al.* (2001) observed blood oxygenation level-dependent (BOLD) signal changes using high-field functional MRI. Migraine attacks were triggered in patients sensitive to a radial flickering checkerboard stimulus. Inhibition of neuronal activation closely resembling a CSD was observed in the occipital cortex, contralateral to the visual aura. This was accompanied by hyperoxygenation, the contrary of what should be expected in an ischemic process *(Fig. 2)*.

Posterior cortical hypoperfusion

The first measures of regional cerebral blood flow (rCBF), carried out in humans during the 1960s showed that aura was accompanied by a decrease in blood flow in the occipital cortex. It was therefore thought that ischemia was responsible for the positive and negative symptoms of the visual scotoma. Olesen *et al.* published a series of work from 1981 describing the temporal and spatial propagation of this hypoperfusion and suggested that it is the consequence rather than the cause of CSD (Olesen *et al.*, 1981).

Cerebral hypoperfusion persists around the limits of oligemia with a 16 to 53% decrease in rCBF observed by perfusion – and diffusion – weighted MRI (Cutrer *et al.*, 1998). There is no argument in favour of tissue ischemia and PET shows normal oxygen extraction (Andersson *et al.*, 1997). In addition, no diffusion anomalies have been observed in the hypoperfusion's zone (Cutrer *et al.*, 1998). However, if we accept Olesen's hypothesis that hypoperfusion is the direct consequence of a neuronal depression, a complete temporal relationship must exist between clinical aura and oligemia. Much experimental evidence exists however, which contradicts the strict relationship as cortical oligemia and aura often occur separately. Oligemia can occur before aura (Olesen *et al.*, 1990) and may persist after aura during the cephalalgic phase (Cutrer *et al.*, 1998). More importantly, it can occur during an attack of migraine without aura.

Two PET studies have confirmed this possibility. Woods *et al.* (1994) reported a chance observation of a young woman who had experienced a migraine attack without aura during measurements of cognitive activation. A large posterior cortical hypoperfusion was recorded from the beginning of the migraine headache which gradually spread anteriorly throughout successive measurements.

PET investigation in 7 patients during spontaneous migraine without aura showed bilateral occipital hypoperfusion spreading to temporal and parietal regions (Denuelle *et al.*, 2005). This hypoperfusion was noted in the 3 to 4 hours following the onset of symptoms (10.3% decrease in rCBF) and persisted after treatment by sumatriptan 4 to 6 hours after symptom onset (12.3% decrease in rCBF) *(Fig. 3)*.

At least in some individuals therefore, migraine without aura can be accompanied by a posterior cortical hypoperfusion resembling that seen classically in migraine with aura.

Thus, two hypotheses can now be put forward:

– Hypoperfusion is the consequence of a neuronal depression which can sometimes remain clinically silent. However, an asymptomatic CSD is highly improbable because of the high neuronal density found in the occipital cortex. The prolonged duration of the hypoperfusion also seems incompatible with a unique wave of CSD leaving one to imagine successive waves of CSD remaining asymptomatic.

– Hypoperfusion is the result of arteriolar vasoconstriction. This posterior oligemia occurs at the beginning of the migraine attack with or without aura and can, depending on the intensity and/or level of cortical excitability, evoke or not a CSD which would then be responsible for the aura. This vascular phenomenon would be controlled by nuclei found in the brain stem (Lance *et al.*, 1983) *(Fig. 4)*.

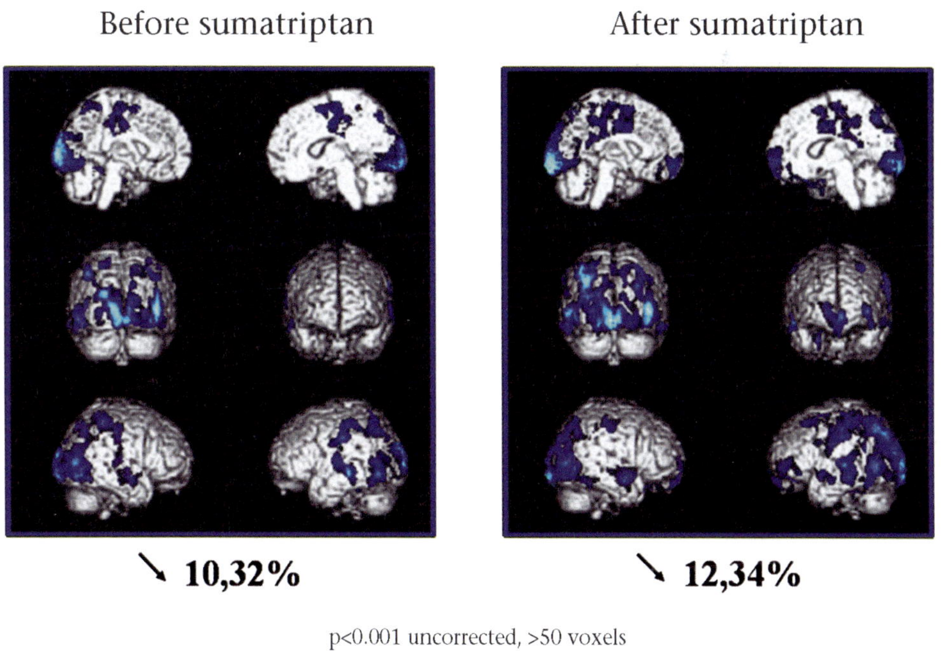

Figure 3. Posterior cerebral hypoperfusion recorded with PET during a spontaneous migraine attack without aura (7 patients). This hypoperfusion was recorded in the first hours of the attack and persisted for up to 4 and 6 hours following the beginning of the attack and relief of pain by tripan injection (Denuelle *et al.* 2008).

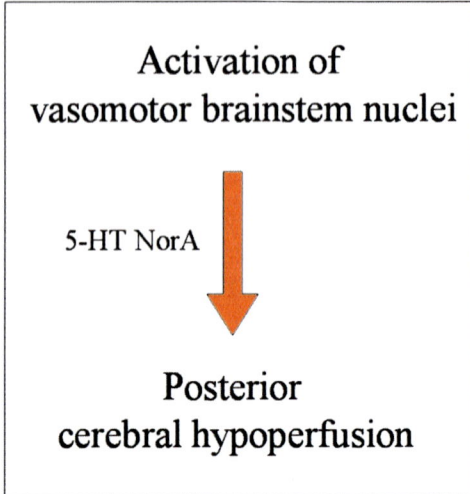

Figure 4. Noradrenergic (locus coeruleus) and serotoninergic (dorsal raphe) nuclei of the brain stem are activated spontaneously or by cortical or subcortical stimulation, evoking vasoconstriction of cortical arteries and spreading oligemia. In predisposed individuals (migrainous terrain), this oligemia facilitates one or more waves of CSD, responsible for the symptoms of aura.

Migraine headache

Present understanding of the mechanisms involved in the migraine headache is based on the physiological anatomy of the trigeminovascular system (TVS) (Goadsby et al., 2002).

Trigeminovascular system

Large blood vessels at the base of the brain, meningeal vessels and dural sinuses are surrounded by a plexus of sensitive nerve fibres from the trigeminal ganglion (1st branch) and, for the posterior cranial fossa, from cervical roots C1-C2.

These primary afferent neurons transmit nociceptive information to second-order neurons located in trigeminal nucleus caudalis and the dorsal horn of the first two cervical segments. This functional neuronal pathway was named the trigeminocervical complex (Moskowitz, 1990) *(Fig. 5)*.

In the rat, activation of this system by electrical stimulation of the trigeminal ganglion evokes the release of vasoactive neuropeptides calcitonin gene related peptide (CGRP), substance P and neurokinin A, which cause a sterile neurogenic inflammation with *(Fig. 6)*:
– vasodilation of meningeal vessels;
– extravasation of plasma proteins;
– degranulation of mast cells;
– platelet activation in capillaries.

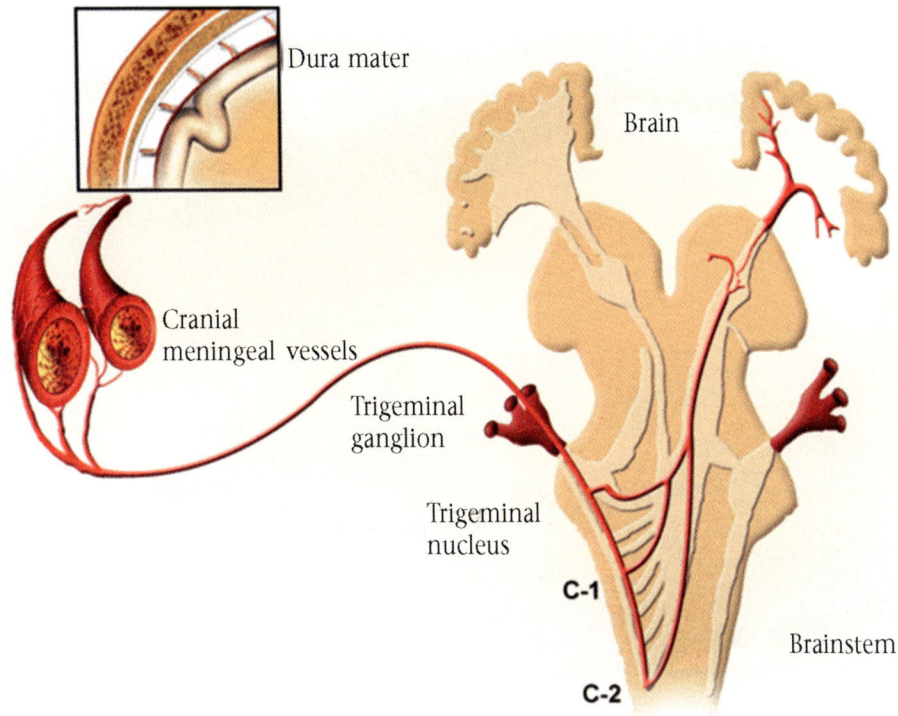

Figure 5. This system consists of 3 components:
– pain-producing cranial meningeal vessels;
– primary afferent neurons which surround these vessels and penetrate the central nervous system *via* the trigeminal ganglion and branches of the first two cervical segments (C1 – C2);
– the trigeminocervical complex (trigeminal nucleus caudalis and dorsal horn at the C1 and C2 levels) functional pathway containing second-order neurons which project on the thalamus and contralateral cortex (Goadsby *et al.*, 2002).

During a migraine attack, mast cell degranulation and platelet activation cause the release of large quantities of serotonin into the cerebral venous system.

Plasma extravasation can be blocked by ergot alkaloids, indomethacin, aspirin and triptans.

Triptans are potent serotonin receptor agonists:
– on 5 HT 1 B receptors which oppose the vasodilation and plasma protein extravasation (PPE) (vasoconstrictor effect);
– on 5 HT 1 D receptors which inhibit vasoactive neuropeptide release *via* trigeminovascular innervation *(Fig. 6)*.

The implication of the TVS in migraine is confirmed by elevated levels of CGRP in the external jugular vein of migraineurs during an attack and their normalization following sumatriptan treatment (Goadsby *et al.*, 1990).

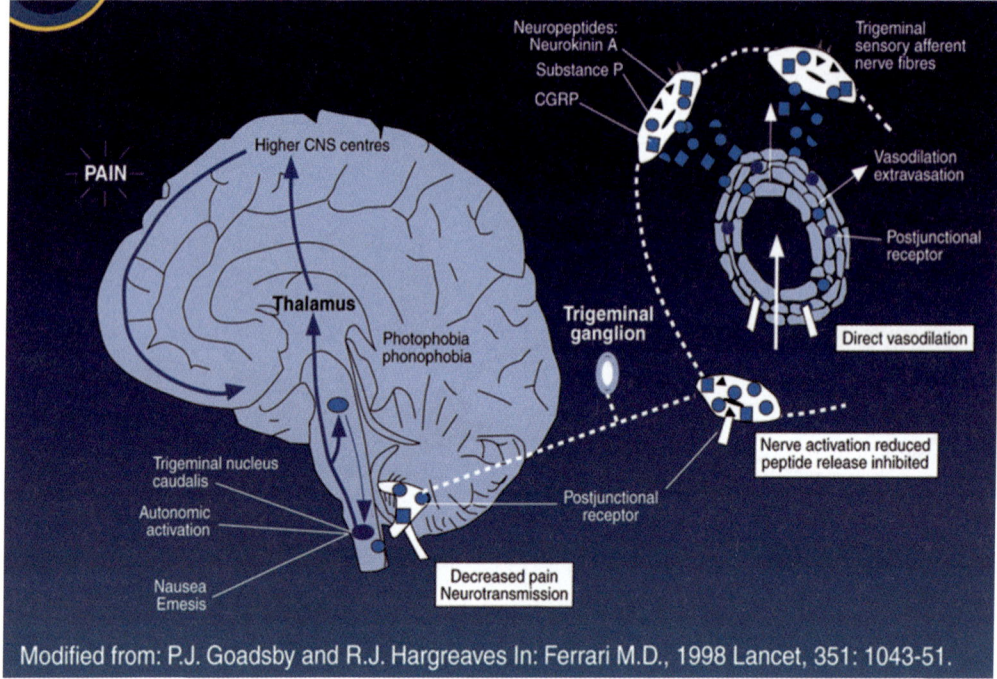

Figure 6. Triptans work peripherally on 5 HT1B receptors which block vasodilation and plasma protein extravasation (vasoconstriction effect) and on 5 HT1D receptors, inhibiting the release of vasoactive neuropeptides. The triptans also work centrally by blocking pain transmission in second-order neurons in the trigeminal nucleus caudalis.

Transmission and central modulation of trigeminal nociception

Electrical or chemical stimulation of the dura mater, the superior sagittal sinus and the trigeminal ganglion evokes the activation of neurons in the superficial layer of the trigeminal nucleus caudalis and in the dorsal horn of the first two cervical segments. Pretreatment by triptan or ergotamine blocks this effect. These substances can work peripherally or within the trigeminal nucleus.

Second-order neurons of the trigeminal pathway project to other brain stem nuclei (nucleus of the solitary tract) to the hypothalamus, the cerebellum, the limbic cortex and the thalamus (ventrobasal complex, posterior and median thalamus).

Conversely, nociceptive neurons of the trigeminal nucleus caudalis and the dorsal horns of the upper spinal cord can be inhibited by fibres coming from higher structures: rostral part of the vestibular nucleus, nucleus raphe magnus, PAG region, hypothalamus, insular cortex and sensorimotor cortex. GABAergic and enkephalinergic inhibitory interneurons also exist.

Naratriptan, zolmitriptan and likely other triptans, may have a central antinociceptive action, acting like morphine on the system of endogenous control of pain, particularly on serotoninergic neurons of the median and dorsal raphe nuclei.

Peripheral and central sensitization

Clinical and experimental findings that speak in favour of a form of central and peripheral sensitization occuring during the migraine are outlined below:

– Coughing or bending over can increase the pain of an attack or bring back the pain several hours after an attack.

– Hyperesthesia of the scalp and reduced pain threshold, especially ipsilateral to the pain of the attack can persist for up to 4 days following the attack (Drummond, 1987).

– Development of hyperalgesia and cutaneous allodynia during migraine attack, which begins within the referred pain area on the ipsilateral head (79% of patients) but which interestingly extends to the other side of the head and/or forearms in 67% of patients (Burstein et al., 2000).

– Facilitation of the R2 nociception-specific blink reflex during but not outside the migraine attack (Kaube et al., 2002).

The reduced efficacy of antimigraine drugs if given too late can therefore be explained by the development of central sensitization.

Link between migraine aura and headache

In 15 to 20% of migraineurs, the headache is systematically preceded by an aura. However, in the majority of cases, the two phenomena are non-related; migraine without aura, aura without headache, auras before a non migraine headache (cluster headache or tension headache).

Experimentally evoked CSD can trigger a sustained increase in blood flow for 40 minutes in the middle meningeal artery which can be abrogated by unilateral transection of the trigeminal nerve or parasympathetic meningeal efferences (Bolay et al., 2002).

CSD, responsible for the aura, activates peripheral nerve endings of the trigeminovascular system which then activate the trigeminal nucleus in the brain stem. This could then cause a parasympathetic reflex producing vasodilation of meningeal vessels and a resulting headache *(Fig. 7)* (Iadecola, 2002).

Molecular genetics of the migraine

Studies of family inheritance and twin studies are in favour of a joint role of environmental factors and genetics in determining migraine with and without aura, though genetical factors are thought to be more important in migraine with aura (Ducros et al., 2002). This genetical susceptibility is polygenic, meaning that the combined effects of a number of different genes are necessary in determining the disease outcome.

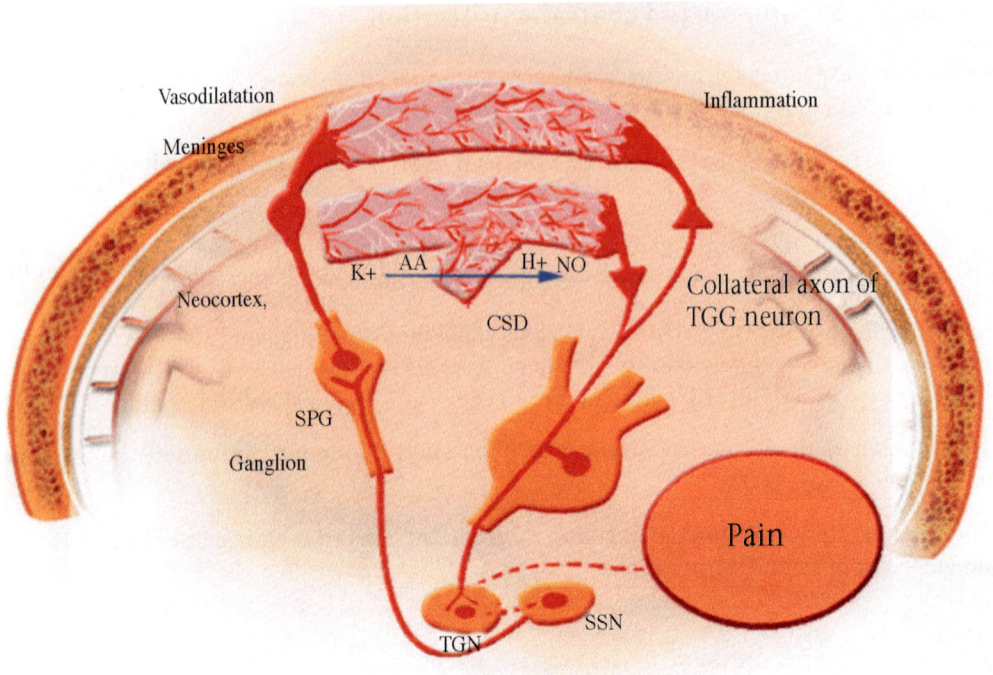

Figure 7. The cortical spreading depression (CSD) releases hydrogen and potassium ions plus other agents including arachidonic acid and nitric oxide in the extracellular space of the neocortex. These agents diffuse towards local blood vessels, depolarising perivascular trigeminal terminals that in turn cause activation of trigeminal nucleus caudalis (TGN) in the brain stem. At the same time, collateral axons of activated neurons in the trigeminal ganglion release pro-inflammatory peptides in the meninges leading to a local inflammatory reaction. The activation of TGN produces vasodilation of meningeal vessels through a parasympathetic pathway originating from the superior salivatory nucleus (SSN) and reaching the meningeal blood vessels *via* the sphenopalatine ganglion (SPG) (Iadecola, 2002).

However, a rare autosomal dominant form of migraine with aura exists, called familial hemiplegic migraine (FHM).

Three genes have been linked to FHM and at least one more gene exists. These three genes code for ion channels and mutations that lead to FHM are suspected to alter neuronal excitability.

The FHM-1 is due to mutations of the *CACNA1A* gene on chromosome 19p13 (Ophoff et al., 1996). This gene codes for the alpha-1A subunit of $Ca_v2.1$ (P/Q) type voltage-gated Ca^{2+} channels which modulate the release of neurotransmitters (noradrenaline, dopamine, acetylcholine, CGRP...). Different mutations of *CACNA1A* are associated with a large number of neurological illnesses from those of episodic form with no permanent anomalies (pure hemiplegic migraine, periodic ataxia, epilepsy) to more severe diseases with permanent, progressive cerebellar ataxia or fatal cerebral oedema. Transgenic mice, carriers of 2 different FHM-1 mutations, express higher neurotransmitter release, particularly cortical glutamate, and a reduced activation threshold of CSD.

The FHM-2 is due to mutations of the gene *ATP1A2* on chromosome 1q23 (De Fusco et al., 2003). This gene, mostly expressed in the glia, codes for the alpha-2 subunit of the transmembrane sodium pump Na^+-K^+ ATPase. Mutations of this gene can lead to many diverse clinical manifestations: pure hemiplegic migraine, epilepsy and more rarely hemiplegic migraine with permanent ataxia, infant hemiplegia and mental retardedness. Mutations lead to a reduction in glutamate and potassium reuptake leading to a build-up in the synaptic cleft which likely increases neuronal excitability.

The FHM-3 is due to mutations of the gene *SCNA1* on chromosome 2q24. This gene codes for voltage-dependent sodium channels and until now, only one mutation has been electrophysiologically analyzed: its presence increases neuronal excitability.

In the migraine without aura, or with non-hemiplegic aura, multiple loci have been found on different chromosomes but none have been formally identified. These data are thus still to be confirmed and it would then be necessary to identify which genes are implicated within each loci.

The sensitivity to the CSD could be the common denominator of the migraine attack. In FHM, mutations of 3 different forms of ion transporters (two neuronal channels and one glial pump) have the same consequence; increase in potassium and glutamate in the synaptic cleft which results in neuronal hyperexcitability and a reduced activation threshold of CSD.

References

- Afridi S, Groadsby PJ. New onset migraine with a brain stem cavernous angioma. *J Neurol Neurosurg Psychiatry.* 2003; 74: 680-2.

- Andersson JLR, Muhr C, et al. Regional cerebral blood flow and oxygen metabolism during migraine with and without aura. *Cephalalgia* 1997; 17: 570.

- Bolay H, et al. Intrinsic brain activity triggers trigeminal meningeal afferents in a migraine model. *Nature Med* 2002; 8: 136-42.

- Burstein R, Curter MF, Yarnitsky D. The development of cutaneous allodynia during a migraine attack. *Brain* 2000; 123: 1703-9.

- Curtrer FM, Sorensen AG, Weisskoff RM, et al. Perfusion-weighted imaging defects during spontaneous migrainous aura. *Ann Neurol* 1998; 43: 25-31.

- Denuelle M, Fabre N, Payoux P, et al. Brainstem and hypothalamic activation in spontaneous migraine attacks: a PET study. *Headache* 2007; 47: 1418-26.

- Denuelle M, Fabre N, Payoux P, et al. Posterior cortical hypoperfusion during spontaneous attacks of migraine without aura: a PET study. *Cephalalgia* 2008; 28: 856-62.

- De Fusco M, Marconi R, Silvestri L, et al. Haploinsufficiency of ATP1 A2 encoding the NA+/K+ pump alpha2 subunit associated with familial hemiplegic migraine type 2. *Nat Genet* 2003; 33: 192-6.

- Ducros A, Tournier-Lasserve E, Bousser MG. The genetics of migraine. *Lancet Neurology* 2002; 1: 285-93.

- Drummond PD. Scalp tenderness and sensitivity to pain in migraine and tension headache. *Headache* 1987; 27: 45-50.

- Goadsby PJ, Lipton RB, Ferrari MD. Migraine-current understanding and treatment. *N Engl J Med* 2002; 346: 257-70.

- Goadsby PJ, Edwinsson L, Ekman R. Vasoactive peptide release in the extra-cerebral circulation of man and the cat during activation of the trigeminovascular system. *Ann Neurol* 1990; 23: 193-6.

- Hadjikhani N, *et al*. Mechanisms of migraine aura revealed by functional MRI in human visual cortex. Proc *Natl Acad Sci* 2001: 4687-92.

- Iadecola C. From CSD to headache: a long winding road. *Nature Med* 2002; 8: 110-2.

- Kaube H, Katsarava Z, Przywara S. Acute migraine headache possible sensitization of neurons in the spinal trigeminal nucleus. *Neurology* 2002; 58: 1234-8.

- Lance JW, Lambert GA, Goadsby PJ, Duckworth JW. Brainstem influences on the cephalic circulation: experimental data from cat and monkey of relevance to the mechanism of migraine. *Headache* 1983; 23: 258-65.

- Lashley KS. Pattern of cerebral integrations indicated by migrainous scotomas. *Arch Neur* 1941; 46: 339.

- Leao AP. Speading depression of activity in cerebral cortex. *J Neurophysiol* 1944; 7: 359-90.

- Milner PM. Note on a possible correspondence between the scotomas of migraine and spreading depression of Leao. *Electroenceph Clin Neurophysiol* 1958; 10: 705.

- Moskowitz MA. Basic mechanisms in vascular headache. *Neurol Clin* 1990; 8: 801-15.

- Olesen J, Larsen B, Lauritzen M. Focal hyperemia followed by spreading oligemia and impaired activation of CBF in classic migraine. *Ann Neurol* 1981; 9: 344-52.

- Olesen J, Friberg L, Olsen TS, *et al*. Timing and topography of cerebral blood flow, aura and headache during migraine attacks. *Ann Neurol* 1990; 28: 791-8.

- Ophoff RA, Terwindt GM, Vergouwe MN, *et al*. Familial hemiplegic migraine and episodic ataxia type-2 are caused by mutations in the Ca(2+) channel gene CACNL1A4. *Cell* 1996; 87: 543-52.

- Rasking NH, Hosobuchi Y, Lamb S. Headache may arise from perturbation of brain. *Headache* 1987; 27: 416-20.

- Weiller C, May A, Limmroth V, *et al*. Brain stem activation in spontaneous human migraine attacks. *Nat Med* 1995; 1: 658-660.

- Wood RP, Jacoboni M, Mazziota JC. Brief report: bilateral spreading cerebral hypoperfusion during spontaneous migraine headache. *N Engl J Med* 1994; 331: 1689-92.

What the epileptologist has to know about the International Headache Society classification of migraine

Anne Donnet
Marseille, France

Introduction to the International Headache Society classification

In 1988, the International Headache Society (IHS) created a classification system that has become the standard for headache diagnosis and research. The first International Classification of Headache Disorders has been translated into 22 languages and galvanized the headache community and stimulated nosologic, epidemiologic, pathophysiologic and genetic research. These criteria facilitated multinational clinical drug trials that have led to the basis of current treatment guidelines.

Fifteen years later, the International Headache Society released the revised and expanded International Classification of Headache Disorders second edition. Like its predecessor, the second edition of the IHS classification separates headache into primary and secondary disorders. The four categories of primary headaches include migraine, tension-type headache, cluster headache and other trigeminal autonomic cephalalgias, and other primary headaches. There are eight categories of secondary headaches: headache attributed to head and/or neck trauma; headache attributed to cranial or cervical vascular disorder; headache attributed to non-vascular intracranial disorder; headache attributed to a substance or its withdrawal; headache attributed to infection; headache attributed to disorder of homoeostasis; headache or facial pain attributed to disorder of cranium, neck, eyes, ears, nose, sinuses, teeth, mouth or other facial or cranial structures; headache attributed to psychiatric disorder. Important changes in the second edition include a restructuring of these criteria for migraine, a new subclassification of tension-type headache, introduction of the concept of trigeminal autonomic cephalalgias, and addition of previously unclassified primary headaches. Several disorders were eliminated or reclassified.

This classification is hierarchical and you must decide how detailed you want to make your diagnosis. The headache disorders are classified into major groups, which are themselves subdivided into levels. In general practice, only the first- or second-digit diagnoses are usually applied while specialist practice and headache specialists would diagnose a more precise diagnostic at the third level. The first digit specifies the major diagnostic type, for example *migraine* (1). The second digit indicates a subtype, for example *migraine with aura* (1.2); the third digit permits more specific diagnosis, for example *typical aura with migraine headache* (1.2.1) or *with non-migraine headache* (1.2.2)... The International Classification of Headache Disorders does not provide a possibility to code for frequency or severity.

IHS Classification of migraine

Migraine is classified into six major categories, the two most important are migraine without aura (1.1) whose criteria are unchanged from 1988, and migraine with aura (1.2).

Migraine without aura (1.1)

Migraine without aura is the most common subtype of migraine. Its criteria are detailed in *Table I* and required at least five attacks, lasting 4 to 72 hours with at least two of four pain features and at least one of two sets of associated symptoms. Criteria are met by various combinations of features *(Table I)*.

Table I. Migraine without aura (1.1)

A. At least 5 attacks fulfilling criteria B-D
B. Headache attacks lasting 4-72 hours (untreated or unsuccessfully treated)

C. Headache has at least two of the following characteristics:
   1. Unilateral location
   2. Pulsating quality
   3. Moderate or severe pain intensity
   4. Aggravation by or causing avoidance of routine physical activity (*e.g.*, walking or climbing stairs)

D. During headache at least one of the following:
   1. Nausea and/or vomiting
   2. Photophobia and phonophobia

E. Not attributed to another disorder

In children, attacks may be shorter, 1 to 72 hours (this may be confirmed with a prospective diary study) and in young children, photophobia and phonophobia may be inferred from their behaviour. Migraine is commonly bilateral in young children; an adult pattern of unilateral pain usually emerges in late adolescence or in early adult life.

When attacks occur on ≥ 15 days/month for 3 months, the diagnoses are both migraine without aura (1.1) and chronic migraine (1.5.1).

Migraine with aura

The IHS criteria for migraine with aura (1.2) have been modified. The typical aura of migraine is characterized by focal neurological features that usually precede migrainous headache. Typical aura symptoms develop over ≥ 5 minutes and last no more than 60 minutes *(Table II)*. The aura consists of fully reversible visual, sensory or language symptoms that precede or accompany the appearance of a migraine-like headache. Both the visual and sensory symptoms often have a bimodal progression with positive symptoms followed by negative symptoms

Typical migraine aura may also occur with non-migrainous headache (1.2.2) *(Table III)*. Lastly, typical aura occurring in the absence of any headache is coded typical aura without headache (1.2.3).

Table II. Typical aura with migraine headache (1.2.1)

A. At least 2 attacks fulfilling criteria B-D

B. Aura consisting of at least one of the following, but no motor weakness:
  1. Fully reversible visual symptoms including positive features (*e.g.*, flickering lights, spots or lines) and/or negative features (*i.e.*, loss of vision)
  2. Fully reversible sensory symptoms including positive features (*i.e.*, pins and needles) and/or negative features (*i.e.*, numbness)
  3. Fully reversible dysphasic speech disturbance

C. At least two of the following:
  1. Homonymous visual symptoms and/or unilateral sensory symptoms
  2. At least one aura symptom develops gradually over ≥ 5 minutes and/or different aura symptoms occur in succession over ≥ 5 minutes
  3. Each symptom lasts ≥ 5 and ≤ 60 minutes

D. Headache fulfilling criteria B-D for 1.1 *Migraine without aura* begins during the aura or follows aura within 60 minutes
E. Not attributed to another disorder

Table III. Typical aura with non-migraine headache (1.2.2)

Typical aura consisting of visual and/or sensory and/or speech symptoms.
Gradual development, duration no longer than one hour, a mix of positive and negative features and complete reversibility characterise the aura which is associated with a headache that does not fulfil criteria for 1.1.

Motor weakness led to the diagnosis of hemiplegic migraine. Two types of hemiplegic migraine are recognized by the IHS. They include familial (FHM) (1.2.4) in which at least one first or second degree relative had had similar attacks or sporadic (1.2.5) in which no first- or second-degree relative with hemiplegic migraine attacks has been identified. FMH is the first migraine syndrome to be linked to a specific set of genetic polymorphism. The criteria of FHM include those of migraine with aura (except that aura include hemiparesis and may last more than 60 minutes) and at least one first or second degree relative with hemiplegic migraine attacks *(Table IV)*. Symptoms of brainstem dysfunction and changes in level of consciousness is coded basilar migraine (1.2.6) *(Table V)*. Because 60% of patients with FHM have basilar-type symptoms, this diagnosis should be coded only when weakness is absent. The headache meets also criteria for migraine without aura.

Table IV. Familial hemiplegic migraine (1.2.4)

A. At least 2 attacks fulfilling criteria B and C
B. Aura consisting of fully reversible motor weakness and at least one of the following: 　1. Fully reversible visual symptoms including positive features (*e.g.*, flickering lights, spots or lines) and/or negative features (*i.e.*, loss of vision) 　2. Fully reversible sensory symptoms including positive features (*i.e.*, pins and needles) and/or negative features (*i.e.*, numbness) 　3. Fully reversible dysphasic speech disturbance
C. At least two of the following: 　1. At least one aura symptom develops gradually over ≥ 5 minutes and/or different aura symptoms occur in succession over ≥ 5 minutes 　2. Each aura symptom lasts ≥ 5 minutes and < 24 hours 　3. Headache fulfilling criteria B-D for 1.1 *Migraine without aura* begins during the aura or follows onset of aura within 60 minutes
D. At least one first- or second-degree relative has had attacks fulfilling these criteria A-E
E. Not attributed to another disorder

Table V. Basilar-type migraine (1.2.6)

A. At least 2 attacks fulfilling criteria B-D
B. Aura consisting of at least two of the following fully reversible symptoms, but no motor weakness: 　1. Dysarthria 　2. Vertigo 　3. Tinnitus 　4. Hypacusia 　5. Diplopia 　6. Visual symptoms simultaneously in both temporal and nasal fields of both eyes 　7. Ataxia 　8. Decreased level of consciousness 　9. Simultaneously bilateral paraesthesias
C. At least one of the following: 　1. At least one aura symptom develops gradually over ≥ 5 minutes and/or different aura symptoms occur in succession over ≥ 5 minutes 　2. Each aura symptom lasts ≥ 5 and ≤ 60 minutes
D. Headache fulfilling criteria B-D for 1.1 *Migraine without aura* begins during the aura or follows aura within 60 minutes
E. Not attributed to another disorder

Probable migraine

A substantially number of patients with features of migraine fail to meet all criteria for migraine without (1.6.1) or with aura (1.6.2). If a single criterion is missing, the proposed code is probable migraine. Epidemiological studies demonstrate that probable migraine is a frequent, undertreated, sometimes disabling disorder.

Childhood periodic syndromes that are commonly precursors of migraine

Three conditions are described: cyclical vomiting (1.3.1); abdominal migraine (1.3.2); benign paroxysmal vertigo of childhood (1.3.3). Cyclical vomiting *(Table VI)* is characterized by recurrent and stereotyped episodes of intense but unexplained nausea and vomiting which last 1 hour to 5 days in children free of symptoms interictally. Abdominal migraine *(Table VII)* is defined as recurrent attacks of abdominal pain associated with anorexia, nausea and sometimes vomiting. Benign paroxysmal vertigo of childhood *(Table VIII)* is a disorder characterized by at least five attacks of severe vertigo resolving spontaneously after minutes to hours. Physical examination and investigations may exclude the other causes of these symptoms.

Table VI. Cyclical vomiting (1.3.1)

A. At least 5 attacks fulfilling criteria B and C
B. Episodic attacks, stereotypical in the individual patient, of intense nausea and vomiting lasting from 1 hour to 5 days
C. Vomiting during attacks occurs at least 4 times/hour for at least 1 hour
D. Symptom-free between attacks
E. Not attributed to another disorder

Table VII. Abdominal migraine (1.3.2)

A. At least 5 attacks fulfilling criteria B-D
B. Attacks of abdominal pain lasting 1-72 hours (untreated or unsuccessfully treated)
C. Abdominal pain has all of the following characteristics: 1. Midline location, periumbilical or poorly localised 2. Dull or "just sore" quality 3. Moderate or severe intensity
D. During abdominal pain at least 2 of the following: 1. Anorexia 2. Nausea 3. Vomiting 4. Pallor
E. Not attributed to another disorder

Table VIII. Benign paroxysmal vertigo of childhood (1.3.3)

A. At least 5 attacks fulfilling criterion B
B. Multiple episodes of severe vertigo, occurring without warning and resolving spontaneously after minutes to hours
C. Normal neurological examination; audiometric and vestibular functions between attacks
D. Normal electroencephalogram

Headache and epilepsy

Given the evidence for increased excitability of neuronal tissue in migraine, parallels with epilepsy are understandable. The IHS classification focuses on three conditions: migraine-triggered seizure, hemicrania epileptica and post-ictal headache.

Migraine and epilepsy

Migraine and epilepsy are comorbid disorders. The criteria for migraine-triggered seizure (1.5.5) require that a seizure fulfilling diagnostic criteria for one type of epileptic attack occurs during or within 1 hour after a migraine aura. This phenomenon is also described as migralepsy.

Headache attributed to epileptic seizure (7.6)

Codes devoted to the link between headache and epilepsy are included in the chapter 7 (headache attributed to non-vascular intracranial disorder). Two conditions are described: hemicrania epileptica (7.6.1) and post-ictal headache (7.6.2) Hemicrania epileptica *(Table IX)* is defined as synchronous ipsilateral headache with migrainous features occurring as an ictal manifestation of the seizure discharge. Diagnosis requires the simultaneous onset of headache with electroencephalographically-demonstrated ictal discharge.

Table IX. Hemicrania epileptica (7.6.1)

A. Headache lasting seconds to minutes, with features of migraine, fulfilling criteria C and D
B. The patient is having a partial epileptic seizure
C. Headache develops synchronously with the seizure and is ipsilateral to the ictal discharge
D. Headache resolves immediately after the seizure

Post-ictal headache with migrainous or tension-type headache features *(Table X)* is a well-recognised consequence of a seizure discharge. Post-ictal headache is often indistinguishable from migraine headache and associated with nausea and vomiting. It is equally common in those with or without a family history of migraine.

It is important for neurologists to familiarize themselves with the diagnostic criteria for the frequently encountered primary headache disorders. However, this revised classification is still evolving and a first revision of this second edition is available on the following link (<www.i-h-s.org>).

Table X. Post-ictal headache (7.6.2): diagnostic criteria

A. Headache with features of tension-type headache or, in a patient with migraine, of migraine headache and fulfilling criteria C and D
B. The patient has had a partial or generalised epileptic seizure
C. Headache develops within 3 hours following the seizure
D. Headache resolves within 72 hours after the seizure

References

1. Headache Classification Subcommittee of the International Headache Society. The International Classification of Headache Disorders, 2nd edition. *Cephalalgia* 2004; 24 (suppl. 1): 1-160.

2. Lipton RB, Bigal ME, Steiner TJ, et al. Classification of primary headaches. *Neurology* 2004; 63: 427-35.

Epilepsy and migraine: a disorder of hyperexcitability?

Geneviève Demarquay[1], Christelle Créac'h[2], Sylvain Rheims[1], Philippe Ryvlin[1]

[1] Lyon, France
[2] Saint-Étienne, France

... I have seen cases intermediate in type between migraine, epileptiform seizures and epilepsy proper
JH Jackson, 1888

Migraine and epilepsy appear as fundamentally different diseases at first sight. However, both of them are characterized by recurrent attacks of nervous system dysfunctions, with a return to baseline between attacks (Haut *et al.*, 2006). They share some clinical characteristics such as trigger factors (visual stimuli, sleep deprivation, stress, menses, etc.), enhanced sensitivity for sensory input such as light and sound and transient neurological symptoms including visual, sensory or speech symptoms. The possible occurrence of migrainous headaches before, during some ictal phases of a partial seizure (hemicrania epileptica) or after any seizure (post-ictal headaches), and the precipitation of an epileptic attack by a typical migrainous aura (migralepsy) also illustrate the reciprocal influences between migraine and epilepsy (De Simone *et al.*, 2007). Moreover, the possible existence of a comorbidity between migraine – especially migraine with aura – and epilepsy (Andermann and Andermann, 1987; Ottman and Lipton, 1994) with a greater severity and frequency of migraine aura in patients who also suffered from epilepsy (Leniger *et al.*, 2003) emphasize the debate of a common pathogenic mechanism that could be related to a state of abnormal neuronal excitability (Lipton *et al.*, 1994). Moreover, an enhanced pathological excitability could explain the therapeutic role of anticonvulsivant drugs in migraine prophylaxis (Welch, 2005; Calabresi *et al.*, 2007; Galetti *et al.*, 2009).

From an experimental point of view, the role of the neuronal excitability has been accepted for a long time in epilepsy but has long been occulted in migraine by the processes of neurogenic inflammation. In the twenty last years, the hypothesis of neuronal excitability was put forward through the development of functional imaging and electrophysiological studies that allowed to analyze *in vivo* the neuronal activity of brain and brainstem during attacks, the role of central sensitization processes leading to cutaneous allodynia, and between attacks and the excitability state between migraine attacks.

The purpose of this review is to present and discuss the alterations of neuronal excitability involved in migraine in order to better understand the similarities but also differences between them.

Alterations of neuronal excitability in epilepsy

Epileptogenesis has been mostly described as a progressive excitation-inhibition imbalance that leads to hyperexcitability of neuronal networks. A large number of different mechanisms leading to this imbalance have been described in epilepsy (Badawy et al., 2009; McCormick and Contreras, 2001). In addition, several of them probably coexist in a single epileptic patient, mainly depending on the underlying anatomical lesion such as, for instance, dysplasia or ischemic insult. Schematically, neuronal hyperexcitability can result from alteration of either intrinsic neurons properties, integration of synaptic inputs or both.

Intrinsic neurons properties are characterized by the balances and fluxes of ion across the membrane and defined the ability of neurons to generate electrical activity (Badawy et al., 2009; McCormick and Contreras, 2001). It has thus been suggested in various animal models that a gradual and sustained membrane depolarization may lead to hyperexcitability (Minkeviciene et al., 2009; Polack et al., 2007; Rheims et al., 2008). A large number of more complex dysfunctions of ion channels have been reported. These so-called channelopathies can originate from both inherited and acquired mechanisms. Indeed, with the development of genetic studies, a large amount of inherited channelopathies have been described in epilepsy, affecting both voltage and ligand gated channel (Helbig et al., 2008; Badawy et al., 2009). Importantly, acquired channelopathies have also been reported. For instance, dysfunctions of A-type potassium channel (Bernard et al., 2004) or hyperpolarization-activated cation channel (Shah et al., 2004) have been described in animal models of temporal lobe epilepsy.

The balance between glutamatergic excitation and GABAergic inhibition may be altered during epileptogenesis. The simplest scheme suggests that this imbalance may be related to a decrease of GABA activity (Sloviter, 1994). However, the role of GABA during epileptogenesis may be much more complex (Cossart et al., 2005; Magloczky and Freund, 2005). Specifically, it has been suggested that GABAergic transmission may switch from inhibition to excitation during epileptogenesis (Ben-Ari and Holmes, 2005). It has indeed been shown in both animal models (Dzhala et al., 2005; Khalilov et al., 2005) and human tissues (Avoli et al., 1999; Cohen et al., 2002) that GABA may act as proconvulsant agent in some situations. Moreover, according to the pivotal role of GABA in the generation of oscillatory activities (Mann and Paulsen, 2007; Beenhakker and Huguenard, 2009), alteration of interneurons activity may lead to the generation of pathological oscillations, as suggested in spike-wave seizures (Steriade, 2005).

Lastly, it should be remembered that non-neuronal and/or non-electrical parameters might also account to hyperexcitability. It has thus been suggested that glia may play a key role during epileptogenesis (Tian *et al.*, 2005). Similarly, the brain metabolic status might also strongly influence networks excitability (Vilchez *et al.*, 2007; Pumain and Laschet, 2006).

Alterations of neuronal excitability in migraine

Alteration in excitability during aura: the role of cortical spreading depression

Clinical findings

Migraine aura occurs in 8 to 30% of the migraine population and consists in focal neurological disturbances that precede or accompany an attack. Most aura symptoms develop over 5 to 20 minutes and usually last less than 60 minutes (Headache Classification Committee, 2004). Aura can manifest itself as visual, sensory, language or motor symptoms and may involve brainstem. Visual aura is the most common form of neurological event and consists of negative symptoms e.g., scotoma, hemianopsia, or of positive symptoms e.g., phosphenes, "fortification spectrum", and less frequently visual distorsions or hallucinations. They move across the visual field, may start at the visual field center and propagate to the peripheral parts, or, sometimes, crossing the midline (Silberstein *et al.*, 2001). In 1941, Lashley analyzed his own visual aura, mapped the trajectory of the scotoma moving across his visual field and deduced that the speed of its spread was more or less 3 mm/min. Milner observed in 1959 that this particular speed of propagation was similar to the cortical spreading depression (CSD) previously described in 1944 in the cerebral cortex of rabbits by Leão (see below).

Cortical spreading depression: an experimental phenomenon

CSD is a self-propagating front of depolarization (corresponding to a slow wave of neuronal hyperexcitability spreading out at a velocity of 3-5 mm/min), followed by a depression of the cortical electrical activity (Gorji, 2001; Smith *et al.*, 2006). This phenomenon can be triggered by a range of several local stimuli, such as electrical, mechanical or chemical cortical stimulations (hypoglycemia, hypoxia or the use of high KCl concentration). The most characteristic electrophysiological feature of CSD is a cortical DC potential transient wave, named the "slow potential change". This electric wave begins with a first small positive component followed by an extracellular negative potential of 5-20 mV lasting 30-50 sec and then by a positive deflection of smaller amplitude but longer duration. This triphasic wave is followed by a depression of normal neuronal activity.

Transient but major changes in cortical ion homeostasis are observed during CSD, marked by a local increase of K+ and glutamate concentration in the extracellular space and an intracellular entry of Ca^{2+}, Na+ and Cl-. The accumulation of K+ in the interstitial space is supposed to cause neuronal depolarization and thus to contribute to the initiation of CSD. The spread of CSD would involve some interactions between astrocytes and neurons, leading to the release and the diffusion of K+ and glutamate into the extracellular space. Ca^{2+} waves may play a role in the initiation and in the modulation of CSD.

Is cortical spreading depression the underlying mechanism of migraine aura?

Earlier neuroimaging studies showed at the start of the attack, a decrease of cerebral blood flow (CBF) was observed in the posterior part of the cortex followed by a slowly spreading area of abnormal CBF moving into more anterior areas at a rate of 2-3 mm/min (Olesen et al., 1981, 1990). Further studies have described haemodynamic processes that may reflect CSD equivalents during migraine aura (Lauritzen, 1994, Cutrer et al., 1998, Sanchez del Rio et al., 1999; Cao et al., 1999). More recently, using functional magnetic resonance imaging (fMRI), Hadjikhani et al. (2001) observed at the initial state of a visual aura (scintillations in the visual field) an increase in the mean BOLD signal which developed sequentially along consecutive regions of calcarine cortex, and retinotopically related to the visual phenomenon. These findings were interpreted as an initial cortical hyperemia lasting a few minutes followed by a long-lasting mild hypoperfusion. Some electrophysiological correlates to CSD were recorded in humans in magnetoencephalography studies that showed a cortical desynchronization in patients experiencing visual aura (Bowyer et al., 2001; Hall et al., 2004). Despite these studies, the occurrence of CSD in the human brain remained long disputed, because of the difficulty to record directly CSD in the human brain *in vivo*. Recently – ten years after a preliminar work by Mayevsky in 1996 – Fabricius et al. (2006) evidenced the existence of CSD *in vivo* in acutely brain-injured patients by electrocorticography. They recorded stereotyped slow potential changes and spreading depressions that propagated with a speed similar to that of Leao's CSD. Finally, the suppression of CSD by some treatments used for migraine prophylaxis (Ayata et al., 2006) is an additional argument suggesting that transient disorders of cortical excitability similar to CSD play a key role in the genesis of migraine aura. Interestingly, among the available antiepileptic drugs used in migraine prophylaxis, some of them – such as lamotrigine – seem to prevent migraine with aura but not migraine without aura (Lampl et al., 1999).

Can cortical spreading depression trigger the rest of the attack?

Aura is usually followed by a migraine headache and is thought by some authors to trigger the rest of the attack. Animal studies support this hypothesis and show that CSD induces long-lasting blood-flow increase in the middle meningeal artery by neurogenic mechanisms requiring both trigeminal and parasympathetic innervations (Bolay et al., 2002). Moreover, CSD can alter the blood-brain barrier permeability by activating brain matrix metallo-protease 9 (MMP9). According to this theory, CSD could lead to depolarization of the trigeminal afferent loop of the reflex arc and then to brainstem activation (Moskowitz, 2007). In migraine without aura, a CSD elicited from "silent" brain areas could trigger the headache (Bolay and Moskowitz, 2005). Several questions remain however unsolved, such as the nature of the trigger headache when aura follows the headache (although this is a rare phenomenon), the ipsi-or controlateral localization between the clinical aura manifestation and the side of the headache (Goadsby, 2001). Moreover, genetic and electrophysiological studies provide arguments that migraine with and without aura could be separate entities. Whether aura generates the rest of the attacks or is triggered by the same process that is responsible for the headache remains a passionate debate.

Links between channelopathy and cortical spreading depression

Until now, the mechanisms that underlie typical migraine aura in patients remain unknown, even though genetic studies of familial hemiplegic migraine (FHM) have allowed a better understanding of molecular mechanisms that may underlie alterations in cortical excitability and enhanced neuronal susceptibility to CSD initiation. In about 50%, FHM mutations are due to mutations in *CACNA1A*, a voltage-gated Ca^{2+} channel gene (FHM type 1). Voltage-dependent Ca^{2+} channels are key protein structures in neuronal cell membranes and participate in the transduction of electrical signals. Consequences of *CACNA1A* mutations result in a "gain of function" with modification of the density and the gating properties of P/Q currents (Ducros *et al.*, 2002). In animal studies, "knock-in" mice carrying FHM-1 mutation within *CACNA1A* show a reduced threshold for CSD (Van den Maagdenberg *et al.*, 2004). Mutations of the Na+/K+-ATPase pump, identified in FHM2, induce a loss of function leading to an increased extracellular concentration of K+ that may trigger CSD. Finally, the mutation of the *SN1A* gene associated with the third subtype of FHM and familial simple febrile seizures alter a voltage-gated sodium channel, resulting in a persistent Na+ influx into neurons (Dichgangs *et al.*, 2005). All the FHM mutations are thought to result in an enhanced glutamate release or a decrease removal of glutamate from the synaptic cleft (Moskowitz *et al.*, 2004), and then to increase susceptibility to CSD.

Alteration in excitability during the migraine attack

Clinical findings

Migraine attack is characterized by a throbbing pain with a worsening after coughing or moving the head and by a hypersensitivity to sensory input such as light, sound or smell. Some patients also present a cutaneous allodynia, defined as a perception of pain resulting from stimulations of skin which are normally painless, within the referred pain area but also outside the ipsilateral head, for instance on the forearms (Burstein *et al.*, 2000). If the characteristics of migraine headaches may reflect a mechanical hypersensitivity of the meningeal primary afferent neurons, periorbital allodynia during migraine attack is thought to reflect sensitization of the trigeminal nucleus caudalis (TNC), which receive both convergent input from meningeal vessels and sensory innervation of the face. Cutaneous allodynia outside the referred pain is considered to reflect a higher order sensitization (third-order thalamic neuronal sensitization) (Burstein, 2001). Moreover, central sensitization of the trigeminocervical complex may also explain the neck pain observed during attacks (Goadsby, 2005).

Experimental data about peripheral and central sensitization from animals to humans

In animal studies, chemical stimulation of the dura induces both activation of afferent neurons in the trigeminal ganglion and an increase of their mechanical sensitivity (Strassman *et al.*, 1996). CSD during migraine aura or other stimulations such as cranial parasympathetic outflow may initiate the peripheral sensitization (Yarnitsky *et al.*, 2003). In migraine, sensitized meningeal nociceptors could lead to the activation and sensitization of second-order central trigeminovascular neurons. Central sensitization is defined as a modulation of nociceptive synaptic transmission leading to facilitated excitatory synaptic reponses and depressed inhibition, thereby amplifying responses to noxious and innocuous inputs (Woolf and Salter, 2000). In migraine, central sensitization is associated with abnormal neuronal excitability in the trigeminal nucleus caudalis (TNC) and involves activation of intracellular signaling cascades and requirement of NMDA receptors (Woolf and Thompson, 1991). A dysfunction of P/Q-type calcium channels in the periaqueductal gray region may contribute to sensitization of the trigeminal pathways (Knight et al., 2002).

In humans, the facilitation of nociceptive blink reflex observed predominantly on the migraine headache side but not in sinusitis support evidence of transient sensitization of neurons in the trigeminal nucleus during acute migraine attacks (Kaube et al., 2002; Katsarava et al., 2002). The enhancement of cortical responses evoked by painful laser stimuli during the migraine may also reflect an hyperexcitability of the cortex that would amplify the central sensitization of pain or a lack of inhibitory control over the transmission of pain to the cortex (de Tommaso et al., 2004).

In conclusion, central sensitization is an important phenomenon thought to play a role in the maintenance and exacerbation of the acute migraine. However, it seems unlikely that the complexity of migraine could be generated by a single process. Other non exclusive hypotheses such as a dysfunction of the pain inhibitory systems located within the brainstem structures are also discussed.

Alteration in excitability in migraine-free period

Clinical findings

Migraine attacks are characterized by a particular sensitivity to visual, auditory external stimuli (Headache Classification Committee, 2004). Some studies suggest that hypersensitivity to external stimuli may persist between migraine attacks. Photosensitivity is the most studied form of interictal hypersensitivity (Main et al., 1997; Vingen et al., 1999; Mulleners et al., 2001), though interictal phonophobia and olfactory hypersensitivity are also observed. Psychophysical studies also showed interictal modifications, such as faster low-level performance in visual processing tasks (Wray et al., 1995). Whereas cutaneous perceptive and nociceptive thresholds are generally considered normal in interictal phase, there may exist some subtle alterations of somato-sensory processes with a reduction in the corneal reflex thresholds and an increased sensitivity to tactile and painful stimulation (Sandrini et al., 2002). During the 15 past years, a lot of electrophysiological studies aimed to investigate interictal cortical information processing in order to better understand the pathophysiology of interictal clinical hypersensitivity in migraine patients. They raised the importance of a loss of habituation during sustained stimulation and debated about the interictal level of cortical excitability.

An interictal lack of habituation

The most reproducible feature observed in migraine patients during the migraine-free period consists in a lack of habituation of evoked and event-related cortical potentials that would be reversible just before and during attacks (Giffin and Kaube, 2002; Schoenen et al., 2003;

Gantenbein and Sandor, 2006). Habituation is a well-known physiological process which consists in a decreased responsiveness by repetition of the same stimuli and which may reflect an adaptative mechanism aimed to protect against sensory overstimulation. The interictal lack of habituation is described for each modality of stimulation, such as vision (Schoenen et al., 1995), audition (Wang et al., 1996; Ambrosini et al., 2001), somato-sensory modality (Siniatchkin et al., 2003) and nociception (Valeriani et al., 2003; de Tommaso et al., 2005). Similar phenomenon is observed with contingent negative variation event-related potentials (Giffin and Kaube, 2002; Schoenen, 2006) and mismatch negativity (de Tommaso et al., 2004). Interestingly, this habituation deficit concerns not only the cortical responses but also some brainstem reflexes such as the nociceptive blink reflex (Di Clemente et al., 2007).

The pathophysiology of this habituation deficit remains unknown, but may be related to an altered serotoninergic transmission. The serotoninergic system plays an important role in the endogenous pain control system and has been implicated in migraine pathophysiology. Serotonin is also known to play a particular role in attentional processes and behavioral habituation. In electrophysiological studies, the high-intensity dependence of auditory-evoked potentials observed in migraine patients is considered to reflect low serotonin transmission (Wang et al., 1996). Moreover, strong intensity dependence of auditory evoked potentials in migraine habituation pattern tends to normalize with fluoxetine prophylaxis, a serotonin reuptake inhibitor (Ozkul and Bozlar, 2002). Another striking feature of interictal habituation deficit in migraineurs is the familial predisposition. Studies show that visual evoked potential habituation and intensity dependence of auditory evoked potential is similar in related parents of migraineurs (Sándor et al., 1999; Siniatchkin et al., 2000). Recently, Di Clemente et al. (2007) also showed that asymptomatic subjects with a first degree migrainous relative show a lack of habituation of the nociceptive blink reflex. This deficient habituation may represent an interictal trait of migraine patients but also en endophenotypic presymptomatic migraine.

Hyper or hypoexcitability of the cortex between attacks?

At first sight, the theory of hyperexcitability described initially in the occipital cortex by Welch in 1990 appeared to fit with the clinical observations of photosensitivity of migraine patients. The increased neuronal density observed in occipital cortex was considered to favor both photophobia and occurrence of CSD. Electrophysiological studies (EEG) had previously showed enhanced photic driving at high frequency in some migraine patients (Golla and Winter, 1959). This phenomenon was called the "H-response" and was confirmed in a later study using the IHS criteria for migraine diagnostic (Chorlton and Kane, 2000). Others EEG findings were observed in migraine patients, such as an increased alpha band phase synchronization to visual stimuli (de Tommaso et al., 2004) and changes in the EEG power spectra during sleep preceding an attack (Goder et al., 2001), suggesting a possible alteration of cortical excitability in these patients. However, the use of transcortical magnetic stimulation (TMS) to assess occipital excitability have also yielded to conflicting results (Giffin and Kaube, 2002; Schoenen et al., 2003; Gantenbein and Sándor et al., 2006). Initially, studies showed decreased thresholds for eliciting phosphenes in migraine patients (Aurora et al., 1998; Mulleners et al., 2001), while an increased phosphene threshold was observed by others (Afra, 1998; Bohotin et al, 2003). In practice, differences in patient selection and differences in stimulation procedure may account for some of discrepancies. Moreover, it seems that thresholds of phosphenes elicited by TMS in migraineurs are too variable and too subjective to be used for the evaluation of occipital excitability (Antal et al., 2006). A second approach to assess cortical excitability relies on the ability to suppress visual perception by using occipital TMS. By using this technique, some authors suggested that an impaired inhibition of cortical activity may explain a cortical hyperexcitability between attacks in migraineurs with aura (Palmer et al., 2000; Chronicle et al., 2006). Conversely, according to a third approach relying on the modulation of EP by repetitive TMS (rTMS), Bohotin showed that the lack of habituation observed between attacks would be associated with a cortical hypoexcitability and would be reversible under high-frequency (10 Hz) rTMS, which are supposed to increase cortical excitability (Bohotin et al., 2002). Conflicting results have also been obtained from motor-evoked potentials in migraine patients for motor threshold, intracortical facilitation and silent period (Giffin and Kaube, 2002; Schoenen et al., 2003).

The question of cortical hypo-or hyperexcitability is also debated regarding the physiopathology of interictal habituation deficit observed in migraineurs. Whether an alteration of cortical inhibitory processes or a decreased preactivation level, possibly to inefficient thalamo-cortical drive (Coppola et al., 2005) could explain the abnormal response to repetitive external stimuli remains unknown (Brighina and Fierro, 2007; Coppola et al., 2007). In all the cases, we must keep in mind the numerous methodological biases that may influence the results obtained among migraineurs: the occurrence of a migraine aura, the frequency of attacks, the duration of prodromal symptoms until 48 hours before attacks, the different kinds of triggers reported by migraineurs.

In conclusion, migraine and epilepsy are two common disorders characterized by recurrent and paroxysmal manifestations of brain dysfunction. Regarding neuronal excitability, the most convincing evidence of a possible continuum is observed for migraine aura, in particular FHM, and epilepsy, with three known mutations associated with enhanced extracellular glutamate concentration resulting in both cortical spreading depression and seizures. However, there seems to be more differences than similarities between the disturbances in neuronal excitability observed in migraine and epilepsy, both during and between attacks. One obvious ictal difference is the propagation speed of cortical spreading depression as compared to that of epileptic discharge (3 mm/min vs. 70-200 mm/s). During the interictal period, epileptiform discharges appear to primarily reflect neuronal hyperexcitability, while the disturbances underlying the abnormal brain function observed in migraine remains unclear. Further studies are certainly warranted to better delineate the complex links between epilepsy and migraine.

References

- Afra J, Mascia A, Gerard P, et al. Interictal cortical excitability in migraine: a study using transcranial magnetic stimulation of motor and visual cortices. *Ann Neurol* 1998; 44: 209-15.

- Andermann E, Andermann F. Migraine-epilepsy relationships: epidemiological and genetic aspects. In: Andermann F, Lugaresi E, ed. *Migraine and epilepsy*. Boston: Butterworth Publishers, 1987: 281-91.

Epilepsy and migraine: a disorder of hyperexcitability?

- Ambrosini A, De Pasqua V, Afra J, et al. Reduced gating of middle-latency auditory evoked potentials (P50) in migraine patients: another indication of abnormal sensory processing? *Neurosci Lett* 2001; 306: 132-4.

- Antal A, Arlt S, Nitsche MA, et al. Higher variability of phosphene thresholds in migraineurs than in controls: a consecutive transcranial magnetic stimulation study. *Cephalalgia* 2006; 26: 865-70.

- Aurora SK, Ahmad BK, Welch KM, et al. Transcranial magnetic stimulation confirms hyperexcitability of occipital cortex in migraine. *Neurology* 1998; 50: 1111-4.

- Avoli, M, Bernasconi, A, Mattia, D, et al. Epileptiform discharges in the human dysplastic neocortex: *in vitro* physiology and pharmacology. *Ann Neurol* 1999; 46: 816-26.

- Ayata C, Jin H, Kudo C, Dalkara T, Moskowitz MA. Suppression of cortical spreading depression in migraine prophylaxis. *Ann Neurol* 2006; 59: 652-61.

- Badawy RA, Harvey AS, Macdonell RA. Cortical hyperexcitability and epileptogenesis: understanding the mechanisms of epilepsy – part 1. *J Clin Neurosci* 2009; 16: 355-65.

- Beenhakker MP, Huguenard JR. Neurons that fire together also conspire together: is normal sleep circuitry hijacked to generate epilepsy? *Neuron* 2009; 62: 612-32.

- Ben-Ari Y, Holmes GL. The multiple facets of gamma-aminobutyric acid dysfunction in epilepsy. *Curr Opin Neurol* 2005; 18: 141-5.

- Bernard C, Anderson A, Becker A, et al. Acquired dendritic channelopathy in temporal lobe epilepsy. *Science* 2004; 305: 532-5.

- Bohotin V, Fumal A, Vandenheede M, et al. Effects of repetitive transcranial magnetic stimulation on visual evoked potentials in migraine. *Brain* 2002; 125: 912-22.

- Bohotin V, Fumal A, Vandenheede M, et al. Excitability of visual V1-V2 and motor cortices to single transcranial magnetic stimuli in migraine: a reappraisal using a figure-of-eight coil. *Cephalalgia* 2003; 23: 264-70.

- Bolay H, Moskowitz MA. The emerging importance of cortical spreading depression in migraine headache. *Rev Neurol* 2005; 161: 655-7.

- Bolay H, Reuter U, Dunn AK, et al. Intrinsic brain activity triggers trigeminal meningeal afferents in a migraine model. *Nature Med* 2002; 8: 136-42.

- Bowyer SM, Aurora KS, Moran JE, et al. Magnetoencephalographic fields from patients with spontaneous and induced migraine aura. *Ann Neurol* 2001; 50: 582-7.

- Brighina F, Fierro B. Cortical hypoactivity or reduced efficiency of cortical inhibition in migraine? *Cephalalgia* 2007; 27: 187-8.

- Burstein R. Deconstructing migraine headache into peripheral and central sensitization. *Pain* 2001; 89: 107-10.

- Burstein R, Yarnitsky D, Goor-Aryeh I, et al. An association between migraine and cutaneous allodynia. *Ann Neurol* 2000; 47: 614-24.

- Calabresi P, Galletti F, Rossi C, et al. Antiepileptic drugs in migraine: from clinical aspects to cellular mechanisms. *Trends Pharmacol Sci* 2007; 28: 188-95.

- Cao Y, Welch KM, Aurora S, Vikingstad EM. Functional MRI-BOLD of visually triggered headache in patients with migraine. *Arch Neurol* 1999; 56: 548-54.

- Chronicle EP, Pearson AJ, Mulleners WM. Objective assessment of cortical excitability in migraine with and without aura. *Cephalalgia* 2006; 26: 801-8.

- Chorlton P, Kane N. Investigation of the cerebral response to flicker stimulation in patients with headache. *Clin Electroencephalogr* 2000; 31: 83-7.

- Coppola G, Vandenheede M, Di Clemente L, et al. Somatosensory evoked high-frequency oscillations reflecting thalamo-cortical activity are decreased in migraine patients between attacks. *Brain* 2005; 128: 98-103.

- Coppola G, Pierelli F, Schoenen J. Is the cerebral cortex hyperexcitable or hyperresponsive in migraine? *Cephalalgia* 2007; 27: 1427-39.

- Cohen I, Navarro V, Clemenceau S, et al. On the origin of interictal activity in human temporal lobe epilepsy in vitro. *Science* 2002; 298: 1418-21.

- Cossart R, Bernard C, Ben-Ari Y. Multiple facets of GABAergic neurons and synapses: multiple fates of GABA signalling in epilepsies. *Trends Neurosci* 2005; 28: 108-15.

- Cutrer FM, Sorensen AG, Weisskoff RM, et al. Perfusion-weighted imaging defects during spontaneous migrainous aura. *Ann Neurol* 1998; 43: 25-31.

- De Simone R, Ranieri A, Marano E, et al. Migraine and epilepsy: clinical and pathophysiological relations. *Neurol Sci* 2007; 28 (Suppl 2): S150-5.

- de Tommaso M, Libro G, Guido M, et al. Habituation of single CO_2 laser-evoked responses during interictal phase of migraine. *J Headache Pain:*. 2005; 6: 195-8.

- de Tommaso M, Guido M, Libro G, et al. Topographic and dipolar analysis of laser-evoked potentials during migraine attack. *Headache* 2004; 44: 947-60.

- de Tommaso M, Guido M, Libro G, et al. Interictal lack of habituation of mismatch negativity in migraine. *Cephalalgia* 2004; 24: 663-8.

- de Tommaso M, Murasecco D, Libro G, et al. Modulation of trigeminal reflex excitability in migraine: effects of attention and habituation on the blink reflex. *Int J Psychophysiol* 2002; 44: 239-49.

- Di Clemente L, Coppola G, Magis D, et al. Interictal habituation deficit of the nociceptive blink reflex: an endophenotypic marker for presymptomatic migraine? *Brain* 2007; 130: 765-70.

- Dichgans M, Freilinger T, Eckstein G, et al. Mutation in the neuronal voltage-gated sodium channel SCN1A in familial hemiplegic migraine. *Lancet* 2005; 5: 371-7.

- Ducros A, Tournier-Lasserve E, Bousser MG. The genetics of migraine. *Lancet Neurol* 2002; 1: 285-93.

- Dzhala VI, Talos DM, Sdrulla DA, et al. NKCC1 transporter facilitates seizures in the developing brain. *Nature Medicine* 2005; 11: 1205-13.

- Fabricius M, Fuhr S, Bhatia R, et al. Cortical spreading depression and peri-infarct depolarization in acutely injured human cerebral cortex. *Brain* 2006; 129: 778-90.

- Galetti F, Cupini LM, Corbelli I, et al. Pathophysiological basis of migraine prophylaxis. *Progress in Neurobiology* 2009: 176-92.

- Gantenbein AR, Sándor PS. Physiological parameters as biomarkers of migraine. *Headache* 2006; 46: 1069-74.

- Giffin NJ, Kaube H. The electrophysiology of migraine. *Curr Opin Neurol* 2002; 15: 303-9.

- Goadsby PJ. Migraine, allodynia, sensitisation and all of that... *Eur Neurol* 2005; 53 (suppl. 1): 10-6.

- Goadsby PJ. Migraine, aura and cortical spreading depression: why are we still talking about it? *Ann Neurol* 2001; 49: 4-6.

- Goder R, Fritzer G, Kapsokalyvas A, et al. Polysomnographic findings in nights preceding a migraine attack. *Cephalalgia* 2001; 21: 31-7.

- Golla FL, Winter AL. Analysis of cerebral responses to flicker in patients complaining of episodic headache. Electroencephalogr *Clin Neurophysiol* 1959; 11: 539-49.

- Gorji A. Spreading depression: a review of the clinical relevance. *Brain Res Brain Res Rev* 2001; 38: 33-60.

Epilepsy and migraine: a disorder of hyperexcitability?

- Hadjikhani N, Sanchez Del Rio M, Wu O, et al. Mechanisms of migraine aura revealed by functional MRI in human visual cortex. *Proc Natl Acad Sci USA* 2001; 10: 4687-92.

- Hall SD, Barnes GR, Hillebrand A, et al. Spatio-temporal imaging of cortical desynchronization in migraine visual aura: a magnetoencephalography case study. *Headache* 2004; 44: 204-8.

- Haut SR, Bigal ME, Lipton RB. Chronic disorders with episodic manifestations: focus on epilepsy and migraine. *Lancet Neurol.* 2006, 5: 148-57.

- Headache Classification Committee. The international Classification of Headache Disorders. *Cephalagia* 2004; S1: 88-101.

- Helbig I, Scheffer IE, Mulley JC, Berkovic SF. Navigating the channels and beyond: unravelling the genetics of the epilepsies. *Lancet Neurol* 2008; 7: 231-45.

- Katsarava Z, Lehnerdt G, Duda B, et al. Sensitization of trigeminal nociception specific for migraine but not pain of sinusitis. *Neurology* 2002; 59: 1450-3.

- Kaube H, Katsarava Z, Przywara S, et al. Acute migraine headache: possible sensitization of neurons in the spinal trigeminal nucleus? *Neurology* 2002; 58: 1234-8.

- Khalilov I, Le Van Quyen M, Gozlan H, Ben-Ari Y. Epileptogenic actions of GABA and fast oscillations in the developing hippocampus. *Neuron* 2005; 48: 787-96.

- Knight YE, Bartsch T, Kaube H, Goadsby PJ. P/Q-type calcium-channel blockade in the periaqueductal gray facilitates trigeminal nociception: a functional genetic link for migraine? *J Neurosci* 2002; 22: RC213.

- Lampl C, Buzath A, Klinger D, Neumann K. Lamotrigine in the prophylactic treatment of migraine with aura: a pilot study. *Cephalalgia* 1999; 19: 58-63.

- Lashley KS. Patterns of cerebral intergration indicated by the scotoma of migraine. *Arch Neurol Psychiatry* 1941; 46: 331-9.

- Lauritzen M. Pathophysiology of the migraine aura. The spreading depression theory. *Brain* 1994; 117: 199-210.

- Leniger T, von den Driesch S, Isbruch K, Diener HC, Hufnagel A. Clinical characteristics of patients with comorbidity of migraine and epilepsy. *Headache* 2003; 43: 672-7.

- Lipton RB, Ottman R, Ehrenberg BL, Hauser WA. Comorbidity of migraine: the connection between migraine and epilepsy. *Neurology* 1994; 44 (10 suppl. 7): S28-32.

- Magloczky Z, Freund TF. Impaired and repaired inhibitory circuits in the epileptic human hippocampus. *Trends Neurosci* 2005; 28: 334-40.

- Main A, Dowson A, Gross M. Photophobia and phonophobia in migraineurs between attacks. *Headache* 1997; 37: 492-5.

- Mann EO, Paulsen O. Role of GABAergic inhibition in hippocampal network oscillations. *Trends Neurosci* 2007; 30: 343-9.

- McCormick DA, Contreras D. On the cellular and network bases of epileptic seizures. *Annu Rev Physi* 2001; 63: 815-46.

- Minkeviciene R, Rheims S, Dobszay MB, et al. Amyloid beta-induced neuronal hyperexcitability triggers progressive epilepsy. *J Neurosci* 2009; 29: 3453-62.

- Mayevsky A, Doron A, Manor T, et al. Cortical spreading depression recorded from the human brain using a multiparametric monitoring system. *Brain Res* 1996; 18: 268-74.

- Milner PM. Note on a possible correspondance between the scotomas of migraine and spreading depression of Leao. *Electroencephalogr Cli Neurophysiol* 1959; 10: 705.

- Moskowitz MA. Pathophysiology of headache – past and present. *Headache* 2007; 47: S58-S63.

- Moskowitz MA, Bolay H, Dalkara T. Deciphering migraine mechanisms: clues from familial hemiplegic migraine genotypes. *Ann Neurol* 2004; 55: 276-80.

- Mulleners WM, Chronicle EP, Palmer JE, et al. Visual cortex excitability in migraine with and without aura. *Headache* 2001; 41: 565-72.

- Olesen J, Larsen B, Lauritzen M. Focal hyperemia followed by spreading oligemia and impaired activation of rCBF in classic migraine *Ann Neurol* 1981; 9: 344-52.

- Olesen J, Friberg L, Olsen TS, et al. Timing and topography of cerebral blood flow, aura, and headache during migraine attacks. *Ann Neurol* 1990; 28: 791-8.

- Ottman R, Lipton RB. Is the comorbidity of epilepsy and migraine due to a shared genetic susceptibility? *Neurology* 1994: 44: 2105-10.

- Ozkul Y, Bozlar S. Effects of fluoxetine on habituation of pattern reversal visually evoked potentials in migraine prophylaxis. *Headache* 2002; 42: 582-7.

- Palmer JE, Chronicle EP, Rolan P, Mulleners WM. Cortical hyperexcitability is cortical under-inhibition: evidence from a novel functional test of migraine patients. *Cephalalgia* 2000; 20: 525-32.

- Polack PO, Guillemain I, Hu E, et al. Deep layer somatosensory cortical neurons initiate spike-and-wave discharges in a genetic model of absence seizures. *J Neurosci* 2007; 27: 6590-9.

- Pumain R, Laschet J. A key glycolytic enzyme plays a dual role in GABAergic neurotransmission and in human epilepsy. *Crit Rev Neurobiol* 2006; 18: 197-203.

- Rheims S, Represa A, Ben-Ari Y, Zilberter Y. Layer-specific generation and propagation of seizures in slices of developing neocortex: role of excitatory GABAergic synapses. *J Neurophysiol* 2008; 100: 620-8.

- Sanchez-Del-Rio M, Reuter U, Moskowitz MA. New insights into migraine pathophysiology. *Curr Opin Neurol* 2006; 19: 294-8.

- Sanchez del Rio M, Bakker D, Wu O, et al. Perfusion weighted imaging during migraine: spontaneous visual aura and headache. *Cephalalgia* 1999; 19: 701-7.

- Sandrini G, Proietti Cecchini A, Milanov I, et al. Electrophysiological evidence for trigeminal neuron sensitization in patients with migraine. *Neurosci Lett* 2002; 317: 135-8.

- Sandor PS, Afra J, Proietti-Cecchini A, et al. Familial influences on cortical evoked potentials in migraine. *Neuroreport* 1999; 10: 1235-8.

- Shah MM, Anderson AE, Leung V, et al. Seizure-induced plasticity of h channels in entorhinal cortical layer III pyramidal neurons. *Neuron* 2004; 44: 495-508.

- Schoenen J, Ambrosini A, Sandor PS, et al. Evoked potentials and transcranial magnetic stimulation in migraine: published data and viewpoint on their pathophysiologic significance. *Clin Neurophysiol* 2003; 114: 955-72.

- Schoenen J, Wanf W, Albert A, Delwide PJ. Potentiation instead of habituation characterized visual evoked potentials in migraine patients between attacks. *Eur J Neurol* 1995; 2: 115-22.

- Silberstein SD, Saper JR, Freitag FG. Migraine: Diagnosis ans Treatment. In: Silbertein SD, Lipton RB, Dalessio DJ (ed) *Wolff's headache and other head pain*. Oxford: Oxford University Press, 2001.

- Siniatchkin M, Kropp P, Gerber WD. What kind of habituation is impaired in migraine patients? *Cephalalgia* 2003; 23: 511-8.

- Siniatchkin M, Kropp P, Neumann M, et al. Intensity dependence of auditory evoked cortical potentials in migraine families. *Pain.* 2000; 85: 247-54.

- Sloviter RS. The functional organization of the hippocampal dentate gyrus and its relevance to the pathogenesis of temporal lobe epilepsy. *Ann Neurol* 1994; 35: 640-54.

- Smith JM, Bradley DP, James MF, Huang CL. Physiological studies of cortical spreading depression. *Biol Rev Camb Philos Soc* 2006; 81: 457-81.

- Steriade M. Sleep, epilepsy and thalamic reticular inhibitory neurons. *Trends Neurosci* 2005; 28: 317-24.

- Strassman AM, Raymond SA, Burstein R. Sensitization of meningeal sensory neurons and the origin of headaches. *Nature* 1996; 384: 560-4.

- Tian GF, Azmi H, Takano T, *et al*. An astrocytic basis of epilepsy. *Nat Med* 2005; 11: 973-81.

- Valeriani M, de Tommaso M, Restuccia D, *et al*. Reduced habituation to experimental pain in migraine patients: a CO(2) laser evoked potential study. *Pain* 2003; 105: 57-64.

- van den Maagdenberg AM, Pietrobon D, Pizzorusso T, *et al*. A CACNA1A knockin migraine mouse model with increased susceptibility to cortical spreading depression. *Neuron* 2004; 4: 701-10.

- Vilchez D, Ros S, Cifuentes D, *et al*. Mechanism suppressing glycogen synthesis in neurons and its demise in progressive myoclonus epilepsy. *Nat Neurosci* 2007; 10: 1407-13.

- Vingen JV, Sand T, Stovner LJ. Sensitivity to various stimuli in primary headaches: a questionnaire study. *Headache* 1999; 39: 552-8.

- Wang W, Timsit-Berthier M, Schoenen J. Intensity dependence of auditory evoked potentials is pronounced in migraine: an indication of cortical potentiation and low serotonergic neurotransmission? *Neurology* 1996; 46: 1404-9.

- Wray SH, Mijovic-Prelec D, Kosslyn SM. Visual processing in migraineurs. *Brain* 1995; 118: 25-35.

- Welch KM. Brain hyperexcitability: the basis for antiepileptic drugs in migraine prevention. *Headache* 2005; 45 (suppl. 1): S25-S32.

- Welch KM, D'Andrea G, Tepley N, *et al*. The concept of migraine as a state of central neuronal hyperexcitability. *Neurol Clin* 1990; 8: 817-28.

- Woolf CJ, Salter MW. Neuronal plasticity: increasing the gain in pain. *Science* 2000; 288: 1765-9.

- Woolf CJ, Thompson SW. The induction and maintenance of central sensitization is dependent on N-methyl-D-aspartic acid receptor activation; implications for the treatment of post-injury pain hypersensitivity states. *Pain* 1991; 44: 293-9.

- Yarnitsky D, Goor-Aryeh I, Bajwa ZH, *et al*. 2003 Wolff Award: possible parasympathetic contributions to peripheral and central sensitization during migraine. *Headache* 2003; 43: 704-14.

Epilepsy and migraine: clinical phenomenology and co-occurrence of symptoms

Carmen Barba, Renzo Guerrini
Firenze, Italy

Epidemiology

Epilepsy and migraine are common chronic disorders, characterized by recurrent neurologic attacks, variously accompanied by headache as well as by gastrointestinal, autonomic, and psychologic features. Differentiating migraine from epilepsy can be difficult in some patients, although the epidemiological profile between epilepsy and migraine is quite different.

The overall incidence of epilepsy in industrialized countries is 25-50 per 100,000 per year, with a highest incidence in the very young (100-200 per 100,000 per year) and in the elderly (100-200 or more per 100,000 per year). Prevalence studies indicate an overall rate of five to six per 1,000 (Hauser *et al.*, 1993; Bell and Sander, 2001). Epilepsy has a relatively constant prevalence rate across industrialized nations and geographic locations. The prevalence of migraine is highest in the Americas and Europe, intermediate in Africa, and lowest in Asia (Scher *et al.*, 1999). Finally, the prevalence of migraine is inversely related to socioeconomic status, a pattern also seen in epilepsy (Burneo *et al.*, 2005; Scher *et al.*, 1999).

The incidence of migraine with aura peaks between ages 12 and 13 years in women (14.1 per 1,000 person per year), whereas migraine without aura peaks between ages 14 and 17 years (18.9 per 1,000 person years). Boys show an early age at onset of migraine with aura (6.6 per 1,000 per year at 5 years of age), with a consequent higher prevalence of migraine than in girls.

The substantial sex differences reported for migraine are relatively smaller for epilepsy (Christensen *et al.*, 2005; Lipton *et al.*, 2001). Although women with epilepsy often show catamenial patterns, hormonal effects are less of a risk factor for epilepsy per se than a precipitant of attacks. Conversely, in women, cyclic hormonal factors are thought to contribute to the excess risk of migraine beginning at the age of menarche, as well as of individual migraine attacks (Lipton *et al.*, 2001).

Migraine and epilepsy are highly comorbid; individuals with either disorder are more than twice as likely to develop both and the increased risk of migraine is evident in every subgroup of epilepsy as defined by age at onset, seizure type, etiology and family history of epilepsy in first-degree relatives (Lipton et al., 1994; Ottman and Lipton, 1996). Ottman and Lipton (1996) assessed the association between migraine and epilepsy in adults and found the prevalence of migraine to be 24% among probands with epilepsy, and 26% in relatives of probands with epilepsy. In the control group of relatives without epilepsy, only 15% had migraine. The prevalence of epilepsy in people with migraine varies from 1% to 17%, with a median of 5.9%, which is substantially higher than the population prevalence of epilepsy (Andermann and Andermann, 1987).

Three alternative models have been proposed to account for the comorbidity of migraine and epilepsy. One possibility is a simple unidirectional causal explanation. However, if migraine were to cause epilepsy by inducing, for example, brain ischemia and injury, the incidence of migraine would be expected to increase before, but not after, the onset of epilepsy. Alternatively, epilepsy might cause migraine by activating the trigeminovascular system, in which one would expect an excess risk of migraine after, but not before, the onset of epilepsy. Since there is an excess risk of migraine both before and after epilepsy onset, a simple unidirectional causal model has been rejected. A second possibility is that shared environmental risk factors might explain this comorbidity. Because the risk of migraine is significantly increased in people with idiopathic or cryptogenic epilepsy, known environmental risk factors cannot account for all of the comorbidity. Ottman and Lipton (1996) tested a third possibility, which is based on the hypothesis of a shared genetic susceptibility and compared risks of migraine in relatives of probands with genetic *versus* nongenetic forms of epilepsy using two proxy measures of genetic susceptibility: a family history of epilepsy in first degree relatives and idiopathic/cryptogenic (*versus* postnatal symptomatic) epilepsy. They also assessed the risk of epilepsy in relatives of epilepsy probands with migraine *versus* that of those without. Neither of these two tests confirmed the hypothesis of a shared genetic susceptibility to migraine and epilepsy.

Finally, Ottman and Lipton (1996) proposed that an altered brain state (increased excitability), might increase the risk of developing both migraine and epilepsy. Enhanced neuronal hyperexcitability and reduced attack threshold are often postulated in the pathophysiologic models of migraine and epilepsy. Reduction in brain magnesium or perturbations in neurotransmitter systems may provide a basis for these alterations in brain excitability. In theory, both genetic and environmental factors could produce these alterations (Bigal et al., 2003).

Recently, Parisi et al., (2008) hypothesized that several etiological factors (either environmental or genetic), such as Na+-K+ ATPase pump impairment, converging on a common final pathway, represented by neuronal membrane hyperexcitability, might manifest as either epilepsy or headache/migraine, or both.

Temporal association between migraine and epilepsy symptoms

In patients with epileptic seizures, headache can occur as an interictal, preictal, ictal, or postictal symptom. Preictal, peri-ictal and, especially, postictal headache may have the clinical characteristics of migraine without aura as well as of tension-like headache (Leniger et al., 2001). Whether the high incidence of migraine or migraine-like manifestations in patients with epileptic seizures relates to the propensity to spreading depression, to the distribution of neurotransmitter activity or to other factors remains speculative (Andermann, 2000).

Interictal headache is defined as not temporally related to seizures. In the series of Leniger *et al.*, (2001) 76.9% of patients with seizure associated migraine and interictal migraine reported identical symptoms in the two situations. In particular, these authors found identical aura symptoms before seizures or migraine attacks in 7 out of 62 patients with seizure independent migraine. Also Marks and Ehrenerg (1993) described 13 (16.5%) of 79 patients with epilepsy and migraine with identical aura symptoms in both disorders.

Preictal and ictal headaches are often neglected, because the seizure overshadows the headache for both the patient and the physician. Particularly, preictal headache is not mentioned in the International Classification of Headache Disorders (ICHD-II, 2004) and has only rarely been reported accurately (Foredrreuther *et al.*, 2002; Yankovsky *et al.*, 2005b). Using a standardized interview, Yankovsky *et al.*, (2005b) described preictal headache in 11 patients with intractable focal epilepsy. Headache was frontotemporal, and ipsilateral to the side of seizure origin in nine out of ten patients with temporal lobe epilepsy (TLE). According to this finding, experimental manipulation of the pia near the circle of Willis and near the tentorium induces pain, usually referred to the ipsilateral temporal and retro-orbital areas. However, preictal headache was contralateral in one patient with TLE and in one with frontal lobe seizures. It was supposed by the authors that contralateral pain in these patients might have been related to unilateral stimulation of the dura over the convexities, which has been shown to produce bilateral or contralateral pain, probably through bilateral termination of the dural nerves near the midline. All seizure-free patients stopped having preictal headache, suggesting that a seizure-free state has a positive influence on any headache in patients with temporal lobe epilepsy.

Peri-ictal headache was more likely to be ipsilateral to seizure onset in TLE than in ETE (extra-temporal epilepsy) also in a study of 100 patients with partial epilepsy (Bernasconi *et al.*, 2001).

Ictal headaches can occur with seizures as the sole or predominant clinical manifestation (Palmini *et al.*, 1992). Headache has been described as a sole manifestation in a child with non-convulsive status epilepticus (Ghofrani *et al.*, 2007). In a large series from an epilepsy unit, 23 of 858 patients experienced ictal pain; 11 of them (1.3%) had headache (Young and Blume, 1983) that was depicted as throbbing by two patients and as sharp or steady by the remaining nine. In the series of Karaali-Savrun (2002), three patients who suffered from ictal headache described their symptoms as localized to their forehead, mild to moderate in severity, lasting for 30-60 seconds, throbbing in nature in two patients and steady in one. Cephalic pain was described in two further patients with parietal lobe epilepsy (Siegel *et al.*, 1999) and it was documented by stereo-EEG (Isler *et al.*, 1987) as hemicranial attacks of pain coincided with seizure activity and lasted seconds to minutes. This phenomenon was defined as "hemicrania epileptica" (Isler *et al.*, 1987) a term that, according to the ICDH-II (2004), is now used to define a rather uncommon condition that can be diagnosed when a migrainous headache lasting seconds to minutes occurs, ipsilaterally to the epileptic discharge, during a partial seizure. An electroencephalographic demonstration of the synchronicity and the ipsilaterality of both manifestations is required.

Most studies had focused on the postictal headache, which can complicate either partial or generalised seizures and is the most frequent headache type associated with epilepsy, with an incidence of 37 to 51% (Ito et al., 2004, Yankovsky et al., 2005a). The frequency of postictal headache is typically high in occipital and temporal lobe epilepsy. Most patients describe it as frontotemporal and strictly unilateral (Yankovsky et al., 2005a). It may present with tension-type features but can be indistinguishable from a true migraine, especially in migrainous patients. The ICDH-II (2004) criteria for postictal headache require the onset of pain within 3 hours after a seizure and its resolution within 72 hours.

At times, headache may be initiated by the premonitory brain events of epilepsy. Likewise, a seizure may be triggered by a migraine aura, a phenomenon which has been called migralepsy, an old term deriving from migra(ine) and (epi)lepsy for "a seizure that may be a composite of symptoms encountered in epilepsy and migraine". Rates of migralepsy reported in populations with comorbid migraine and epilepsy range from 1.7 to 16% (Marks and Ehrenberg, 1993; Velioglu and Ozmenoglu, 1999). ICDH-II criteria (2004) for this condition require: (A) migraine fulfilling criteria for migraine with aura; (B) a seizure fulfilling diagnostic criteria for one type of epileptic attack occurring during or within 1 hour after a migraine aura. However, only a few case reports have been published and most of these have been considered genuine occipital seizures imitating migraine aura and "migralepsy" as an erroneous diagnosis (Panayiotopoulos, 1999; 2006). Misdiagnosis of visual seizures as migraine with visual aura is frequent (Guerrini et al., 1998) even if elementary visual hallucinations of occipital seizures are fundamentally different from the visual aura of migraine. In occipital seizures, elementary visual hallucinations are usually the first and often the only ictal symptom and may multiply and increase in size in the course of the seizure and progress to other occipital and extraoccipital manifestations and convulsions. They are stereotyped for each patient, usually lasting for seconds, and consist of mainly multiple, bright coloured, small circular and rotating spots, circles, or balls. Mostly, they appear in a temporal hemifield often moving contralaterally or in the centre where they may be flashing. Blindness often occurs from the beginning. Postictal headache, often indistinguishable from migraine, is common. It often occurs 3-15 min after the seizure ends, a situation known in migraine as the "asymptomatic interval" (end of migraine aura to the onset of headache). Migraine-like attacks prompted by occipital seizures have been defined as the "epilepsy-migraine sequence" (Panayiotopoulos, 2005; 2006).

In migraine, the visual aura usually starts as a flickering, uncolored, zigzag line in the center of the visual field and affects the central vision. It gradually progresses over > 4 minutes, usually lasting < 30 minutes, towards the periphery of one hemifield, often leaving a scotoma. The total duration of visual auras is 60 minutes. Acute onset of visual aura is very rare. Furthermore, the visual aura of migraine rarely has a daily frequency; nonvisual ictal occipital symptoms, such as eye and head deviation and repetitive eyelid closures, do not occur; it is probably exceptional to progress to nonvisual epileptic seizures.

Less typical features of the visual migraine aura, such as spots, circles and beads, with or without colors, have been reported (Shevell, 1996), but usually they are non dominant; clustering of other symptoms, as reported above, betrays their migraine nature.

Migraine-triggered seizures have particularly been associated with basilar-type migraine and catamenial epilepsy (Laplante et al., 1983). Basilar-type migraine is characterized by a aura often lasting less than 1 hour indicating focal dysfunction of the brainstem, the occipital lobes, or both, and is usually followed by severe, throbbing occipital headache and vomiting. A hemianopic field disturbance can rapidly expand to involve both visual fields, leading, at times, to temporary blindness that may precede the other symptoms. If present and marked, the alterations in consciousness define confusional migraine. Basilar-type migraine may be difficult to differentiate from complex partial seizures and from the postictal state. In one instance, an episode that was interpreted as an attack of basilar artery migraine triggered by photic stimulation was captured by EEG (Swanson and Vick, 1978). The characteristics of the recorded episode are actually consistent with those of a typical occipital seizure triggered by photic stimulation.

In a large series of patients with epilepsy, it has been reported that 3% of those also having migraine, experienced seizures during or immediately following a migraine aura (Marks and Ehrenberg, 1993). Patients with catamenial epilepsy and patients with migraine with aura were at increased risk for an association between these two disorders. Similar findings were described by Velioglu and Ozmenoglu (1999) who found a direct relationship between migraine and epilepsy (a migraine-induced epilepsy) in 1.7% of their patients (seven patients) with seizures. Patients were at increased risk for both conditions if they had migraine with aura and catamenial epilepsy.

Clinical characteristics of occipital epileptic seizures and their differential diagnosis from migraine attacks

Ictal discharges originating in the occipital cortex may remain localized or spread to adjacent areas. Ictal recordings clearly show that spreading may be either rapid or remarkably slow and can occur after many minutes of discharge limited to the occipital lobe (Naquet et al., 1987; Aso et al., 1988). Hemiclonic seizures or complex partial seizures can then occur, and secondary generalization is frequent. Infrasylvian propagation to mesiotemporal limbic structures is frequent and accompanied by automatisms typical of temporal lobe epilepsy (Bancaud et al., 1961; Takeda et al., 1969; Williamson et al., 1992). The patients' ability to recall visual symptoms points to initial localization of the ictal discharge near the calcarine fissure, followed by slow propagation to adjacent areas. When the discharge is occipitotemporal at the onset, visual phenomena cannot usually be recalled (Munari et al., 1993).

Visual phenomena are the initial ictal manifestation in all patients able to describe their symptoms. These are usually described as bright, colorful or multicolored rings or spots which are fixed or flashing in the periphery of the visual field, rotating or moving slowly to the opposite half-field (Davidson and Watson, 1956; Ricci and Vigevano, 1993; Guerrini et al., 1994, 1995). Some patients report ictal blindness or severe blurring of vision, limited to one hemifield or involving the entire visual field, usually after the positive visual phase but occasionally as the first symptom (Aso et al., 1988; Maeda et al., 1990). A minority of patients describe complex visual phenomena such as micropsia (Dulac et al., 1986) or viewing "shadow people", accompanied by a frightened feeling (Shuper and Vining, 1991). A vague feeling of fear may be an isolated manifestation, or be accompanied by epigastric discomfort without visual phenomena. The latter ictal pattern suggests that in rare patients, visual stimuli may precipitate seizures in which the discharge initiates in the limbic areas (Benbadis et al., 1996; Isnard et al., 1998). Visual phenomena are often followed by a versive phase, with "conscious" head and eye deviation most frequently towards the side of the initial visual symptoms but occasionally contralaterally (Guerrini et al., 1995).

When the discharge spreads outside the occipital cortex, the most frequent ictal pattern is a sequence of epigastric discomfort, unresponsiveness, and vomiting. Fleeting sharp abdominal pain is sometimes reported before clouding of consciousness (Guerrini et al., 1994, 1995) or early during the attack (Davidson and Watson, 1956; Walker et al., 1995). Oroalimentary automatisms may occur late in the seizure. Postictal headache is frequent and is often reported in patients with ictal headache but the ictal and postictal pain are usually reported to have different characteristics (Guerrini et al., 1995).

Misdiagnosis of occipital seizures with migraine and vice versa is common, especially in the pediatric age. A common mistake is that of not recognizing visual induced seizures since, in a number of patients, they are strictly stimulus related and, as such, may be occasional and lack the typical tendency to recurrence, which is considered the hallmark of epilepsy. Two main factors may contribute to make differential diagnosis difficult. The clinical features of occipital seizures are often subtle and similarities with migraine symptoms can be very close (Panayiotopoulos, 1987; Guerrini et al., 1995). The symptom cluster of visual aura, abdominal discomfort, vomiting, and headache can make clinical differentiation between occipital seizures and migraine particularly difficult. Some authors have suggested that when visual disturbances are the only manifestation of a seizure, the differentiation between migraine and epilepsy depends mainly on the rapidity of their onset and disappearance (Deonna, 1988). The same could apply to ictal vomiting associated with reduced awareness (Wilson, 1992). A comparison of the elementary visual hallucinations of migraine and of epileptic seizures showed that seizures are predominantly characterized by circular or spherical multicolored patterns, as opposed to the predominantly black and white ictal patterns of migraine (Panayiotopoulos, 1994). Rapid onset and resolution of the visual disturbance would be more in keeping with an epileptic seizure (Deonna, 1988): prolonged attacks with nausea and vomiting preceded by visual aura and accompanied by altered consciousness, rather than by complete unresponsiveness, would indicate migraine (Wilson, 1992). Nevertheless, these distinctions can be misleading because spread of the discharge from the occipital cortex can be very slow and responsiveness may be maintained while the patient is vomiting (Guerrini et al., 1994).

In patients with visually triggered occipital seizures and infrequent attacks, it can be difficult to recognize the triggering role of TV, computer screens, or bright lights. This occurs especially if the slow spread of ictal activity causes overt symptoms to appear when the patient is not looking at the provoking stimulus.

Epileptic syndromes, migraine and migraine-like seizures (Table I)

Migraine and migraine-like seizures may be features of certain syndromes, such as idiopathic childhood occipital epilepsy and rolandic epilepsy of childhood. Idiopathic occipital epilepsy is a clinical syndrome, initially described by Gastaut, with onset between 15 months and 17 years, mainly characterized by initial visual symptoms followed by ictal manifestations consistent with ictal spread to extraoccipital areas, including hemiclonic seizures, automatisms, dysphasia, dysesthesia and adversative manifestations (Gastaut, 1982). Seizures are predominantly diurnal and may be frequent. EEG typically shows occipital paroxysms activated by eye closure and with fixation-off sensitivity (Panayiotopoulos, 1989). However, in some there may only be random occipital spikes or occipital spikes only in sleep EEG or transient activation of typical EEG

Table I. Clinical characteristics of idiopathic epilepsy syndromes often associated with migraine or migraine-like seizures (modified by Covanis, 2006)

	Early onset idiopathic childhood occipital epilepsy	Rolandic epilepsy of childhood	Late onset – idiopathic childhood occipital epilepsy	Idiopathic photosensitive occipital lobe epilepsy
Mean age at onset (range), y	4-5 (1-15)	7-8 (1-15)	10-11 (4-17)	15 (5-17)
Male/female ratio	1	1.5	1	0.7
Main seizure symptoms at onset	Emesis and/or other autonomic disturbances	Facial sensorimotor, speech arrest	Elementary visual hallucinations or blindness	Elementary visual symptoms, epigastric discomfort, headache, version, vomiting
Common duration of seizures	9 min	1-3 min	Seconds to 1 min	20 seconds to 25 minutes
Circadian distribution (%)	Nocturnal (64)	Nocturnal (70)	Diurnal (100)	Depending on trigger
Focal nonconvulsive status epilepticus (30 min), %	40	Exceptional	Exceptional	Relatively frequent
Common interictal EEG spike location	Multifocal	Centrotemporal	Occipital	Occipital
Onset of ictal EEG	Posterior or anterior brain regions	Lower part of pre and post central gyrus	Occipital	Occipital
Prognosis	Excellent	Excellent	Unpredictable: 70% remit	Closely related to photosensitivity range

abnormalities *(Fig. 1)* (Guerrini *et al.*, 1997b). A positive family history of migraine, was found in patients from several series of children with idiopathic occipital epilepsy (Beaumanoir and Jeckiel, 1987; Gastaut and Zifkin, 1987). Following a seizure, approximately 25 to 40% of patients develop migraine-like headaches (Gastaut, 1982; Panayiotopoulos, 1989). Headache mainly orbital, may also be ictal, preceding the visual or other seizure symptoms in a small number of patients (Covanis *et al.*, 2005).

A well defined subgroup of children with an early onset variant of idiopathic occipital epilepsy has been characterized, in which seizures are often prolonged and autonomic symptoms prominent (Covanis, 2006). Autonomic seizures consist of episodes of disturbed autonomic function, often accompanied by emesis. Other autonomic manifestations include pallor (or, less often, flushing or cyanosis), mydriasis (or, less often, miosis), cardiorespiratory and thermoregulatory alterations, incontinence, hypersalivation, and modifications of intestinal motility. More conventional seizure symptoms often appear after the onset of autonomic manifestations. The child, who is initially fully conscious, becomes confused and unresponsive. Eyes turn to one side or gaze widely open. Only half of the seizures end with brief hemiconvulsions or generalized convulsions. Headache or, more often, cephalic auras and behavioral disturbances may

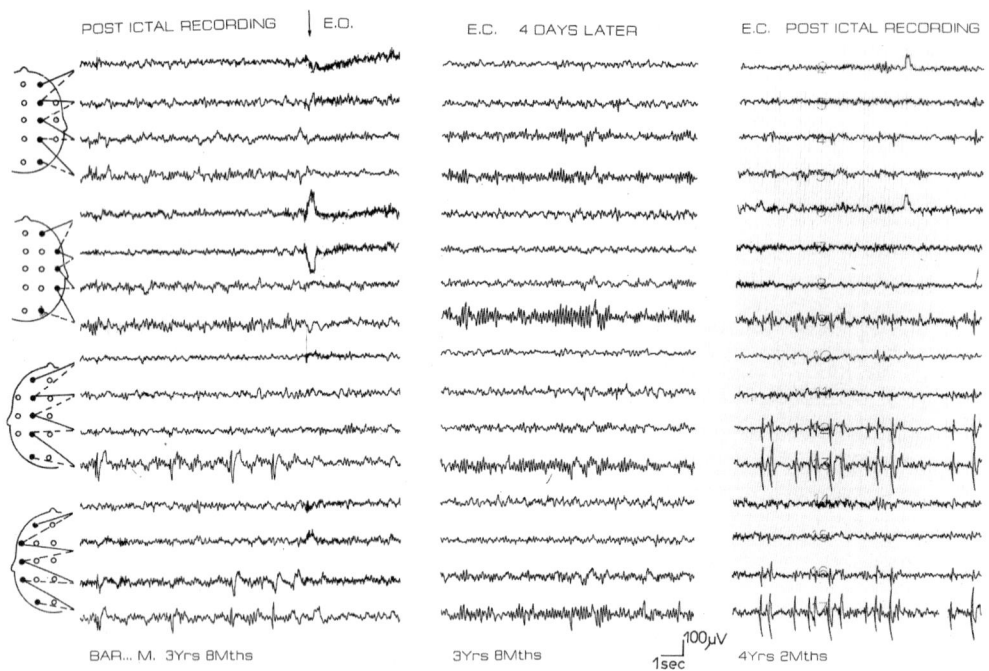

Figure 1. Idiopathic occipital epilepsy of childhood.
Left: at age 3 years and 8 months, 2 hours after a seizure, presence of spikes and spikes and waves on the left occipital region blocked by eyes opening.
Middle: EEG is normal four days later.
Right: at age 4 years and 2 months, postictal EEG still shows very frequent spikes on the left occipito-temporal posterior region.
E.O: eyes open; E.C: eyes closed.

occur, particularly at onset, leading to a misdiagnosis of migraine (Covanis, 2006). The syndrome, often referred to as "Panayiotopoulos syndrome", is conceptualized as "a benign age-related focal seizure disorder occurring in early and mid-childhood". However, since data about long-term follow up and drug discontinuation are scanty, prognostic issues should be expressed cautiously in the individual child.

Several studies pointed out that the incidence of migraine in children with benign rolandic epilepsy was higher than would be expected by chance; however different rates of co-occurrence have been provided by different authors (Kinast et al., 1982; Bladin 1987; Giroud et al., 1989; Septien et al., 1991; Andermann and Andermann, 1992; Ong et al., 1999; Andermann, 2000). Giroud et al. (1989) compared the incidence of migraine in four groups of children: 1) 28 children with absence epilepsy; 2) 42 children with rolandic epilepsy of childhood; 3) 38 children with partial epilepsy; and 4) 30 children with head trauma and assessed that the incidence of migraine in rolandic epilepsy of childhood was higher than the other groups. In 1987, Bladin noted that 20 (67%) of 30 rolandic epilepsy patients had recurrent headaches during the evolution of seizures, and 24 (80%) developed typical migraine after remission of rolandic epilepsy of childhood. Conversely, Santucci et al., (1985) found no significant difference in migraine prevalence between children with benign rolandic epilepsy and healthy controls.

Wirrell et al. (2006) compared the prevalence of migraine in children and their parents in three cohorts: benign rolandic epilepsy, cryptogenic or symptomatic partial epilepsy, and healthy controls, to determine whether migraine was more prevalent in the rolandic epilepsy group. Although they found that migraine tended to be more common in children with epilepsy, the prevalence did not differ when those with rolandic epilepsy were compared to the cryptogenic/symptomatic partial epilepsy group. However, since most children included in the study had had seizures within the preceding year, it was still possible that they would then develop migraine after remission of rolandic epilepsy.

Although seizures with migraine-like characteristics can be observed in patients with a brain lesion ((Guerrini et al., 1994) a much larger category of patients experience, as their main clinical manifestation, recurrent seizures with visual and autonomic symptoms in the context of idiopathic photosensitive occipital lobe epilepsy (IPOE) (Michelucci and Tassinari, 1993; Ricci and Vigevano 1993; Ferrie et al., 1994; Guerrini et al., 1995). Clinical features include seizure onset between ages 4 and 18 years, frequent familial occurrence of similar events or other forms of epilepsy, brief or long-lasting seizures with preferential propagation to the temporal lobe, and a stereotyped seizure pattern in the individual patient *(Fig. 2)*. Secondary generalization occurs in the majority of patients for whom systematic description of seizure patterns was provided (Tassinari et al., 1989; Guerrini et al., 1995). Two patients have been reported in whom, visual-induced occipital seizures began in adolescence, after remission of rolandic epilepsy (Guerrini et al., 1996). Prognosis is generally favorable since seizures can be controlled by monotherapy. Some patients received no drugs and had no seizure recurrence when exposure to the trigger was restricted. However, patients with a wide photosensitivity range may have recurrent seizures despite medical treatment. Nosologically, these findings indicate an age- and localization-related idiopathic epilepsy with a specific mode of precipitation, akin to primary reading epilepsy (Wolf, 1992). The long-term outcome of the disorder is not known since there are no reports of extended follow-up

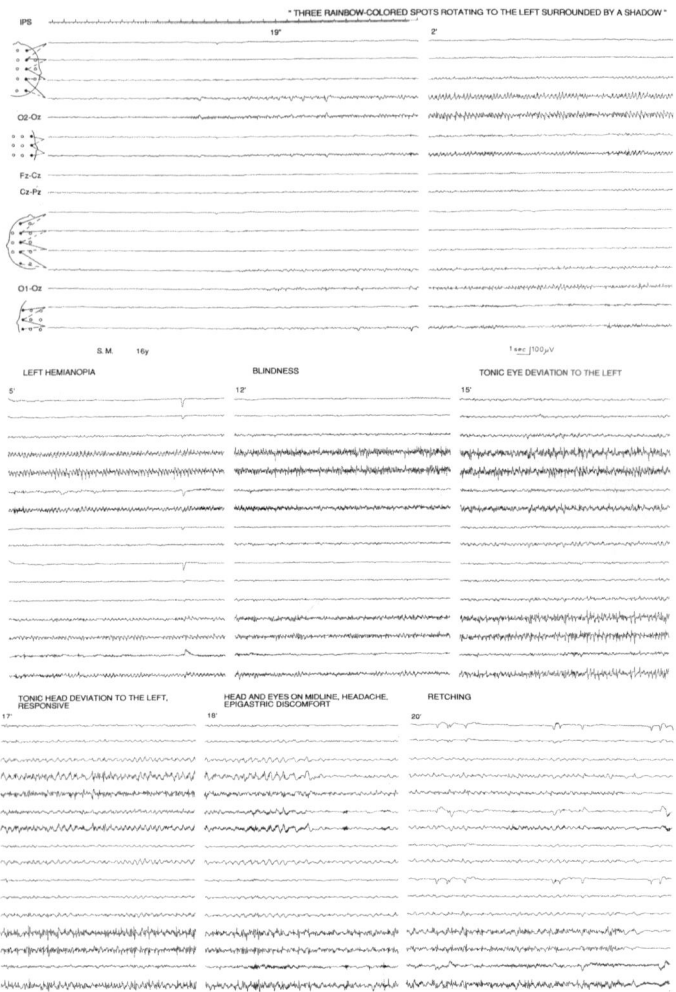

Figure 2. IPS-induced occipital seizure.
Seizure activity begins over the O2-Oz channel. At 19" the patient describes "three rainbow-colored spots surrounded by a dark shadow" in the left visual field that roll to the left. The ictal discharge spreads progressively over the right occipito-posterior temporal area while transmitted waves are present contralaterally (from 2' to 5'); the patient reports the spots have slowly faded while the shadow progressively covers the left visual field, producing left hemianopia. At 12' seizure activity involves both occipito-posterior temporal areas with right predominance; the patient reports complete blindness, as confirmed by visual field assessment. At 15' slow waves are recognisable on the right and the patient's eyes deviate towards the left. At 17' ictal discharge progressively slows to rhythmic spike and slow waves on the right while it persists on the left. The patient shows head deviation towards the left and remains responsive. At 18' the patient's head returns to midline; complains of sudden headache, epigastric discomfort and at 20' retches. Ictal discharge stops on the right hemisphere 18 minutes after seizure onset (18'), but continues for a further 2 minutes on the left (20'). Continuous clinical testing evidenced a gradual postictal improvement of visual blurring. The patient fully recovered vision 3 minutes after the end of the seizure but remained agnosic, and was able to identify objects 6 minutes later.
IPS: intermittent photic stimulation; ": seconds; ': minutes.

after discontinuation of treatment. Considering that this is a form of pure photosensitive epilepsy and that age at onset was not different from that of generalized photosensitivity (Binnie and Jeavons, 1992), it is likely that the seizure susceptibility may persist through adulthood. Background EEG activity is normal in IPOE. Spontaneous interictal spikes or spike and wave complexes are present over the occipital region in most patients, localized to or predominant at the Oz electrode, and associated with generalized spike and wave complexes in some. Abnormalities are enhanced both on eye closure and with the eyes closed. Some patients also have rolandic spikes (Guerrini et al., 1995). A normal interictal EEGs is possibile (Herrlin 1960; Davidoff and Johnson, 1963; Rushton 1981; Glista et al., 1983; Michelucci and Tassinari, 1993). Intermittent photic stimulation (IPS) provokes a photoparoxysmal response that is occipital, generalized or both *(Fig. 3 and 4)*. The photosensitivity range is wide (5-40 Hz), with marked interindividual variability (Guerrini et al., 1995). Some patients show an apparently generalized photoconvulsive response, preceded by paroxysmal occipital driving. However, a photoparoxysmal response is not demonstrable in all patients (De Marco and Ghersini, 1985). In such cases visual evoked responses are often helpful for diagnosis, since in our experience they are always of abnormally high amplitude (Guerrini et al., 1997a).

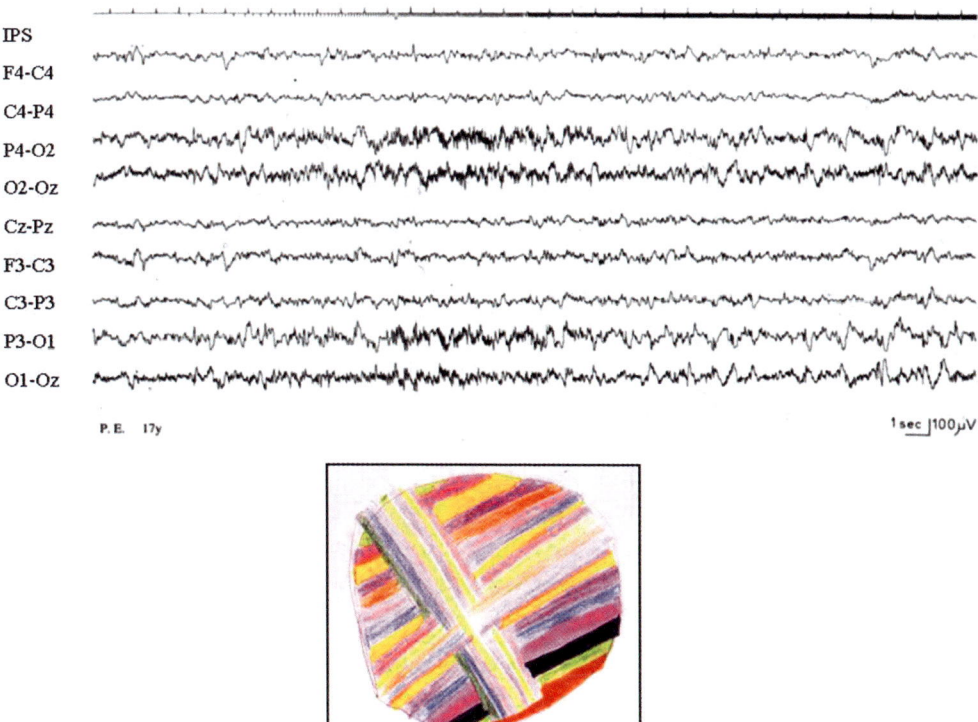

Figure 3. 17 year-old girl with idiopathic photosensitive occipital lobe epilepsy.
Eyes open: A photoparoparoxysmal response is driven by IPS at 30 Hz and is accompanied by visual symptoms which the girl describes as "phosphorescent multicolored spots moving in the visual field".

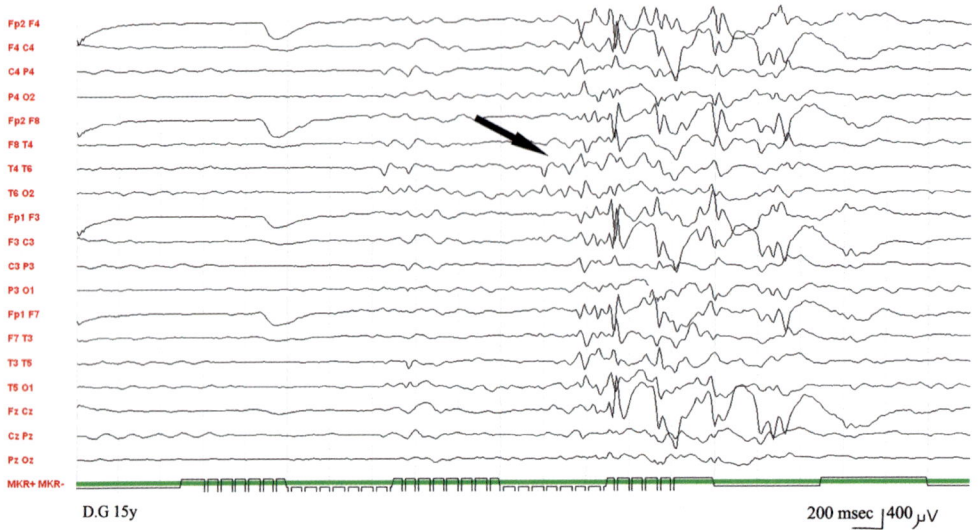

Figure 4. A photoparoparoxysmal response is driven by IPS at 15 Hz.
Note that a short right temporo-occipital discharge precedes the more diffuse EEG abnormalities (black arrow).

Conclusions

Migraine and epilepsy are highly comorbid, although the hypothesis of a shared genetic susceptibility has not been conclusively demonstrated (Ottman and Lipton, 1996). An increased excitability has been hypothesized to underlie the risk of developing both migraine and epilepsy. Increased excitability may be produced by reduction in brain magnesium or perturbations in neurotransmitter systems possibly due to both genetic and environmental factors, such as Na+-K+ ATPase pump impairment (Ottman and Lipton, 1996; Parisi et al., 2008).

In patients with epileptic seizures, headache can occur as an interictal, preictal, ictal, or postictal symptom, making differentiation of migraine from epilepsy difficult in some patients (Leniger et al., 2001). Misdiagnosis of occipital seizures with migraine and *vice versa* is common, especially in the pediatric age (Guerrini et al., 1998) although hallucinations of migraine and of epileptic seizures may show differences in that the latter are predominantly characterized by circular or spherical multicolored patterns, as opposed to the predominantly black and white ictal patterns of migraine (Panayiotopoulos, 1994).

Although seizures with migraine-like characteristics can be observed in patients with a brain lesion (Guerrini et al., 1994), they are most frequently encountered in certain idiopathic epilepsy syndromes. A category of patients experience, as their main clinical manifestation, recurrent seizures with visual and autonomic symptoms in the context of idiopathic photosensitive occipital epilepsy (Guerrini et al., 1995). Some may also exhibit the features of benign rolandic epilepsy (Guerrini et al., 1996). Photic-induced occipital seizures often involve a succession of visual and vegetative symptoms, sometimes with headache. They can be mistaken for migraine, especially if the seizure activity does not spread above the sylvian fissure and there is no recognizable ictal motor activity (Guerrini *et al.*, 1997b). The age-related onset, clinical and EEG characteristics may help differential diagnosis.

References

- Andermann F. Migraine and the benign partial epilepsies of childhood: evidence for an association. *Epileptic Disord* 2000; 2: 37-9.

- Andermann E, Andermann FA. Migraine-epilepsy relationships: epidemiological and genetic aspects. *In:* Andermann FA, Lugaresi E, eds. *Migraine and Epilepsy*. Boston: Butterworths, 1987: 281-91.

- Andermann F, Andermann E. Migraine and epilepsy, with special reference to the benign epilepsies of childhood. *Epilepsy Research* 1992; 6 (suppl.): 207-14.

- Aso K, Watanabe K, Negoro T, *et al.* Photosensitive partial seizure: The origin of abnormal discharges. *J. Epilepsy* 1988; 1: 87-93.

- Bancaud J, Bonis A, Morel P, *et al.* Épilepsie occipitale à expression « rhinencéphalique » prévalente (corrélations électrocliniques à la lumière des investigations fonctionnelles stéréotaxiques). *Rev Neurol* 1961; 105: 219.

- Beaumanoir A, Jekiel M. Electrographic observations during attacks of classical migraine. *In:* Andermann F, Lugaresi E, eds. *Migraine and Epilepsy*. London: Butterworth Heinemann, 1987: 163-80.

- Bell GS, Sander JW. The epidemiology of epilepsy: the size of the problem. *Seizure* 2001; 10: 306-16.

- Benbadis SR, Gerson WA, Harvey JH, Lüders HO. Photosensitive temporal lobe epilepsy. *Neurology* 1996; 46: 1540-2.

- Bernasconi A, Andermann F, Bernasconi N, *et al.* Lateralizing value of peri-ictal headache: A study of 100 patients with partial epilepsy. *Neurology* 2001; 56: 130-2.

- Bigal ME, Lipton RB, Cohen J, Silbersteind SD. Epilepsy and migraine. *Epilepsy Behav* 2003; 4: 13-24.

- Binnie CD, Jeavons PM. Photosensitive epilepsies. *In:* Roger J, Bureau M, Dravet C, Dreifuss FE, Perret A, Wolf P, eds. *Epileptic Syndromes in Infancy, Childhood and Adolescence (2nd edition)*. London: John Libbey and Company, 1992: 299-305.

- Bladin PF. The association of benign rolandic epilepsy with migraine. *In:* Andermann F, Lugaresi E, eds. *Migraine and Epilepsy*. Boston: Butterworths, 1987: 145-52.

- Burneo JG, Tellez-Zenteno J, Wiebe S. Understanding the burden of epilepsy in Latin America: a systematic review of its prevalence and incidence. *Epilepsy Res* 2005; 66: 63-74.

- Christensen J, Kjeldsen MJ, Andersen H, *et al.* Gender differences in epilepsy. *Epilepsia* 2005; 46: 956-60.

- Covanis A, Ferrie CD, Koutroumanidis, *et al.* Panayiotopoulos syndrome and Gastaut type idiopathic childhood occipital epilepsy. *In:* Roger J, Bureau M, Dravet C, Genton P, Tassinari CA, Wolf P, eds. *Epileptic Syndromes in Infancy, Childhood and Adolescence (4th edition)*. Montrouge: John Libbey Eurotext, 2005: 227-53.

- Covanis A. Panayiotopoulos syndrome: a benign childhood autonomic epilepsy frequently imitating encephalitis, syncope, migraine, sleep disorder, or gastroenteritis. *Pediatrics* 2006; 118: 1237-43.

- Davidoff RA, Johnson LC. Photic activation and photoconvulsive responses in a nonepileptic subject. *Neurology* 1963; 13: 617-21.

- Davidson S, Watson CW. Hereditary light sensitive epilepsy. *Neurology* 1956; 6: 235-61.

- De Marco P, Ghersini L. Videogames and epilepsy. *Dev Med Child Neurol* 1985; 27: 519-21.

- Deonna T. Paroxysmal disorders which may be migraine or may be confused with it. In: Hockaday JM, ed. *Migraine in Childhood*. London: Butterworths, 1988: 75-87.

- Dulac O, Chiron C, Valenza A, *et al*. Épilepsie généralisée primaire avec crises partielles. *Boll Lega It Epil* 1986; 54/55: 71-4.

- Ferrie CD, De Marco P, Grunewald RA, *et al*. Video game induced seizures. *J Neurol Neurosurg Psychiatry* 1994; 57: 925-31.

- Föredrreuther S, Henkel A, Noachtar S, Straube A. Headache associated with epileptic seizures: epidemiology and clinical characteristics. *Headache* 2002; 42: 649-55.

- Gastaut H. A new type of epilepsy: benign partial epilepsy of childhood with occipital spike-waves. *Clin Electroenceph* 1982; 13: 13-22.

- Gastaut H, Zifkin BG. The risk of automobile accidents with seizures occurring while driving: relation to seizure type. *Neurology* 1987; 37: 1613-6.

- Ghofrani M, Mahvelati F, Tonekaboni H. Headache as a sole manifestation in nonconvulsive status epilepticus. *J Child Neurol* 2007; 22: 660-2.

- Giroud M, Couillault G, Arnould S, *et al*. Centro-temporal epilepsy and migraine: a controlled study: evidence for a non-fortuitous association. *Pediatrie* 1989; 44: 659-64.

- Glista GG, Frank HG, Tracy FW. Video games and seizures. *Arch Neurol* 1983; 40: 588.

- Guerrini R, Ferrari AR, Battaglia A, *et al*. Occipitotemporal seizures with ictus emeticus induced by intermittent photic stimulation. *Neurology* 1994; 44: 253-9.

- Guerrini R, Dravet C, Genton P, *et al*. Idiopathic photosensitive occipital lobe epilepsy. *Epilepsia* 1995; 36: 883-91.

- Guerrini R, Bonanni P, Parmeggiani L, Belmonte A. Benign partial rolandic epilepsy evolving into idiopathic photosensitive occipital lobe epilepsy. *Epilepsia* 1996; 37: 98.

- Guerrini R, Bonanni P, Parmeggiani L, Belmonte A. Adolescent onset of idiopathic photosensitive occipital epilepsy after remission of benign rolandic epilepsy. *Epilepsia* 1997a; 38: 777-81.

- Guerrini R, Belmonte A, Veggiotti P, *et al*. Delayed appearance of interictal EEG abnormalities in early onset childhood epilepsy with occipital paroxysms. *Brain Dev* 1997b; 19: 343-6.

- Guerrini R, Bonanni P, Parmeggiani L, *et al*. Induction of partial seizures by visual stimulation. Clinical and electroencephalographic features and evoked potential studies. *Adv Neurol* 1998; 75: 159-78.

- Hauser WA, Annegers JF, Kurland LT. Incidence of epilepsy and unprovoked seizures in Rochester, Minnesota, 1935-1984. *Epilepsia* 1993; 34: 453-68.

- Headache Classification Subcommittee of the International Headache Society. The International Classification of Headache Disorders: 2nd edition. *Cephalalgia* 2004; 24: 9-160.

- Herrlin KM. Epilepsy, light sensitivity and left handedness in a family with monozygotic triplets. *Pediatrics* 1960; 25: 385-99.

- Isler H, Wieser HG, Egli M. Hemicrania epileptica: synchronous ipsilateral ictal headache with migraine features. In: Andermann F, Lugaresi E, eds. *Migraine and epilepsy*. Boston: Butterworth, 1987: 249-63.

- Isnard J, Guénot M, Fischer C, *et al*. A stereoelectroencephalographic (SEEG) study of light-induced mesiotemporal epileptic seizures. *Epilepsia* 1998; 39: 1098-103.

- Ito M, Adachi N, Nakamura F, *et al*. Characteristics of postictal headache in patients with partial epilepsy. *Cephalalgia* 2004; 24: 23-8.

- Karaali-Savrun F, Ksan Bg, Yeni S, *et al.* Seizure-related headache in patients with epilepsy. *Seizure* 2002; 11: 67-9.

- Kinast M, Lueders H, Rothner AD, Erenberg G. Benign focal epileptiform discharges in childhood migraine (BFEDC). *Neurology* 1982; 32: 1309-12.

- Laplante P, Saint JH, Bouvier G. Headache as an epileptic manifestation. *Neurology* 1983; 33: 1493-5.

- Leniger T, Isbruch K, von den Driesch S, *et al.* Seizure-associated headache in epilepsy. *Epilepsia* 2001; 42: 1176-9.

- Lipton RB, Ottman R, Ehrenberg BL, Hauser WA. Comorbidity of migraine: the connection between migraine and epilepsy. *Neurology* 1994; 44: 28-32.

- Lipton RB, Stewart WF, Diamond S, *et al.* Prevalence and burden of migraine in the United States: data from the American Migraine Study II. *Headache* 2001; 41: 646-57.

- Marks DA, Ehrenberg BL. Migraine-related seizures in adults with epilepsy, with EEG correlation. *Neurology* 1993; 43: 2476-83.

- Maeda Y, Kurokawa T, Sakamoto K, *et al.* Electroclinical study of video-game epilepsy. *Dev Med Child Neurol* 1990; 32: 493-500.

- Michelucci R, Tassinari CA. Television-induced occipital seizures. *In:* Andermann F, Beaumanoir A, Mira L, Roger J, Tassinari CA, eds. *Occipital Seizures and Epilepsies in Children*. London: John Libbey Eurotext, 1993: 165-71.

- Munari C, Tassi L, Francione S, *et al.* Occipital seizures with childhood onset in severe partial epilepsy: a surgical perspective. *In:* Andermann F, Beaumanoir A, Mira L, Roger J, Tassinari CA, eds. *Occipital Seizures and Epilepsies in Children*. London: John Libbey Eurotext, 1993: 203-11.

- Naquet R, Menini C, Riche D, *et al.* A. Photic epilepsy problems raised in man and animals. *Ital J Neurol Sci* 1987; 8: 437-47.

- Ong HT, Rothner DA, Wyllie E, *et al.* Primary headache disorders in children with benign epileptiform discharges. *Neurology* 1999; 52: 45.

- Ottman R, Lipton RB. Is the comorbidity of epilepsy and migraine due to a shared genetic susceptibility? *Neurology* 1996; 47: 918-24.

- Palmini A, Gloor P. The localizing value of auras in partial seizures: a prospective and retrospective study. *Neurology* 1992; 42: 801-8.

- Panayiotopoulos CP. Fixation-off-sensitive epilepsy in eyelid myoclonia with absence seizures. *Ann Neurol* 1987; 22: 87-9.

- Panayiotopoulos CP. Benign childhood epilepsy with occipital paroxysms: a 15-year prospective study. *Ann Neurol* 1989; 26: 51-6.

- Panayiotopoulos CP. Elementary visual hallucinations in migraine and epilepsy. *J Neurol Neurosurg Psychiatry* 1994; 57: 1371-4.

- Panayiotopoulos CP. Elementary visual hallucinations, blindness, and headache in idiopathic occipital epilepsy: differentiation from migraine. *J Neurol Neurosurg Psychiatry* 1999; 66: 536-40.

- Panayiotopoulos CP. Occipital lobe epilepsies. *In:* Panayiotopoulos CP, ed. *The Epilepsies: Seizures, Syndromes and Management*. Oxford: Bladon Medical Publishing, 2005: 416-29.

- Panayiotopoulos CP. "Migralepsy" and the significance of differentiating occipital seizures from migraine. *Epilepsia* 2006; 47: 806-8.

- Parisi P, Piccioli M, Villa MP, *et al.* Hypothesis on neurophysiopathological mechanisms linking epilepsy and headache. *Med Hypotheses.* 2008; Jan 7.

- Ricci S, Vigevano F. Occipital seizures provoked by intermittent light stimulation: ictal and interictal findings. *J Clin Neurophysiol* 1993; 10: 197-209.

- Rushton DN. Space invader epilepsy. *Lancet* 1981; 1: 501.

- Santucci M, Giovanardi Rossi P, *et al*. Migraine and benign epilepsy with rolandic spikes in childhood: a case-control study. *Dev Med Child Neurol* 1985; 27: 60-2.

- Scher AI, Stewart WF, Lipton RB. Migraine and headache: a meta-analytic approach. *In:* Crombie IK, ed. *Epidemiology of Pain*. Seattle: IASP Press, 1999: 159-70.

- Septien L, Pelletier JL, Brunotte F, *et al*. Migraine in patients with history of centro-temporal epilepsy in childhood: a Hm-PAO SPECT study. *Cephalgia* 1991; 11: 281-4.

- Shevell MI. Acephalgic migraines of childhood. *Pediatr Neurol* 1996; 14: 211-5.

- Shuper A, Vining EPG. Photosensitive complex partial seizures aggravated by phenytoin. *Ped Neurol* 1991; 7: 471-2.

- Siegel AM, Williamson PD, Roberts DW, *et al*. Localized pain associated with seizures originating in the parietal lobe *Epilepsia* 1999; 40: 845-55.

- Swanson JW, Vick NA. Basilar artery migraine 12 patients, with an attack recorded electroencephalographically. *Neurology* 1978; 28: 782-6.

- Takeda A, Bancaud J, Talairach J, *et al*. Epileptic seizures of occipital origin. *Rev Neurol* 1969; 121: 306-15.

- Tassinari CA, Rubboli G, Plasmati R, *et al*. Television-induced epilepsy with occipital seizures. *In:* Beaumanoir A, Gastaut H, Naquet R, eds. *Reflex Seizures and Reflex Epilepsies*. Genève: Éditions Médecine et Hygiène, 1989: 241-3.

- Velioglu SK, Ozmenoglu M. Migraine-related seizures in an epileptic population. *Cephalalgia* 1999; 19: 797-801.

- Walker MC, Smith SJM, Sisodiya SM, Shorvon SD. Case of simple partial status epilepticus in occipital lobe epilepsy misdiagnosed as migraine: clinical, electrophysiological, and magnetic resonance imaging characteristics. *Epilepsia* 1995; 36: 1233-6.

- Williamson PD, Thadani VM, Darcey TM, *et al*. Occipital lobe epilepsy: clinical characteristics, seizure spread patterns, and results of surgery. *Ann Neurol* 1992; 31: 3-13.

- Wilson J. Migraine and epilepsy. *Dev Med Child Neurol* 1992; 34: 645-7.

- Wirrell EC, Hamiwka LD. Do children with benign rolandic epilepsy have a higher prevalence of migraine than those with other partial epilepsies or nonepilepsy controls? *Epilepsia* 2006; 47: 1674-81.

- Wolf P. Reading epilepsy. *In:* Roger J, Bureau M, Dravet C, Dreifuss FE, Perret A, Wolf P, eds. *Epileptic Syndromes in Infancy, Childhood and Adolescence (2nd edition)*. London: John Libbey Company, 1992: 281-98.

- Yankovsky AE, Andermann F, Bernasconi A. Characteristics of headache associated with intractable partial epilepsy. *Epilepsia* 2005a; 46: 1241-5.

- Yankovsky AE, Andermann F, Mercho S, *et al*. Preictal headache in partial epilepsy. *Neurology* 2005b; 65: 1979-81.

- Young GB, Blume WT. Painful epileptic seizures. *Brain* 1983; 106: 537-54.

Differential diagnosis between epilepsy and particular forms of migraine with prolonged neurological symptoms in children

Dominique Parain
Rouen, France

Introduction

The boundaries between migraine and epilepsy are in most cases clearly distinct. Their differentiation may be difficult, especially in children. Although migraine-like symptoms such as visual hallucinations, consciousness disturbances, headache, and vomiting are also common cardinal ictal features in epileptic seizures, the analysis of the occurrence of these symptoms is often sufficient to perform the diagnosis. The progression of symptoms and underlying physiopathological events are very different in these 2 disorders. Progression is usually slow in migraine with aura (MWA) and faster in epilepsy. The differential diagnosis between migraine with typical visual aura and brief occipital seizures have been previously described in the chapter "Migraine and epilepsy: clinical phenomenology and co-occurrence of symptoms".

According to the International Classification of Headache Disorders (ICHD-II) (Headache Classification Subcommittee of the IHS, 2004), the duration of aura in migraine with typical aura (MWTA) is less than 1 hour. The differential diagnosis between migraine and epilepsy may be more difficult in case of attacks with prolonged neurological symptoms (> 1 hour) with a combination in some of the following symptoms: visual, sensory, language disturbances but also decrease the level of consciousness, confusion or agitation. These patients are most often children and usually admitted to the Pediatric Emergency Unit.

The sequences of EEG abnormalities are well known during partial epileptic seizure. In contrast, the EEG remains normal at least during the first hour of migraine aura as in MWTA with a normal duration of aura (Lauritzen *et al.*, 1981). Therefore, EEG is not useful in migraine without aura and in MWTA. In the other types of atypical prolonged migraine aura, EEG abnormalities have been reported during and just after the aura but, until recently, the different types of abnormalities and the temporo-spatial sequence have not been well identified. We will see that the ICHD-II is not well adapted for these pediatric patients with prolonged atypical aura. Currently they could be classified into 3 entities:

1. *Sporadic hemiplegic migraine* (SHM) is an entity recognized by ICHD-II (see Chapter 3) with an aura lasting up to 24 hours with a combination of visual, sensory, speech symptoms frequently associated with unilateral motor weakness. However, in our experience, some patients have the same type of prolonged aura but without motor weakness. These patients, without motor weakness, cannot be easily classified by ICHD-II.

2. *Basilar type migraine* (BTM) is also recognized by ICHD-II (see also Chapter 3). This type of migraine appears most often in children. The aura symptoms originate mainly from the brainstem and frequently last less than 1 hour with ataxia, diplopia, vertigo and followed by headache. According to ICHD-II, BTM is the only type of migraine where a decreased level of consciousness may be observed. In few patients, the aura in BTM may last from several hours up to 2 days and are associated with EEG abnormalities, either occipital slow waves (Lapkin *et al.*, 1977) or diffuse beta activity (Parain and Samson-Dollfus, 1984; Soriani *et al.*, 1996). Occipital spikes and waves may be recorded between attacks of BTM, however, this occurs only in patients with an association of BTM and seizures (Camfield *et al.*, 1978; De Romanis *et al.*, 1996).

3. *Confusional migraine* is not rare in children. This type of migraine was first described by Garcon and Barlow in 1970 in 4 children, between the ages of 8 and 16 years with acute confusional state and agitation lasting 4 to 24 hours associated with headache (Gascon and Barlow, 1970). The EEG during the confusional state had shown diffuse slow waves abnormalities (Emerys, 1977). Minor head trauma may be a trigger for this type of migraine (Haas and Laurie, 1988). This entity is not recognized by ICHD-II, probably because it represents an overlap between SHM and BTM with prolonged aura, even if confusion is not identified as a symptom of one of these two types of atypical aura. Patients with hemiparesis, speech disturbance and confusion would be classified as having SHM and patients with confusion and visual symptoms, ataxia and vertigo would be classified as having BTM.

The site of dysfunction is mainly on one hemisphere in SHM and on the brainstem in BTM. We will attempt to demonstrate that confusion and/or impaired consciousness in migraine are mainly associated with a bi-hemispheric dysfunction and, at a lesser degree, with a brainstem dysfunction. Thus these symptoms are essentially encountered in Bi-Hemispheric Migraine (BHM). This type of migraine has been barely evoked in ICHD-II as a part BTM (bi-hemispheric form of basilar type migraine) even if there are few clues for brainstem dysfunction.

Therefore, this suggests that ICHD-II is not well adapted to classify these children who are admitted to an Emergency Pediatric Unit for prolonged atypical aura. The careful analysis of clinical data may be insufficient to determine the type of migraine aura, the site of dysfunction and to make a definite differential diagnosis as regards epilepsy. Some tests may be useful. The first test, for this purpose, is an EEG. Transcranial Doppler (TCD) and Single Photon Emission Tomography (SPECT) may also be useful tools to evaluate the vascular events associated with the electrical events in migraine aura and to localise the site of dysfunction (Parain *et al.*, 2007). Recently, perfusion MRI has been used to localize the hemodynamic changes during aura (Sanchez del Rio and Alvarez Linera, 2004).

Since 1980, we have investigated, when possible, patients who were admitted to our Pediatric Emergency Unit for atypical prolonged migraine aura. Some of these data have been published (Parain and Samson-Dollfus, 1984; Parain *et al.*, 2007). After the assessment of the entire data, we propose an *electroclinical classification of atypical prolonged migraine with aura* in children (patients with Familial Hemiplegic Migraine – FMH – were not included and the relationship of FMH and epilepsy is described in another chapter). As the classification of epileptic seizures is also based on electro-clinical characteristics (Commission on Classification and Terminology of the ILAE, 1989), this approach could be a useful tool for differential diagnosis between these types of migraine and epileptic seizures. This classification could be also helpful to improve the ICHD-II in this field. ICHD-II is primarily clinical but the collection of sets of well documented patients with clinical and EEG data may be useful to clarify some types of migraine with atypical prolonged aura.

The *electroclinical classification of migraine with atypical prolonged aura* should be divided into 3 groups:
1. prolonged migraine aura lasting 1-24 hours with unilateral EEG slow wave abnormalities;
2. prolonged migraine aura lasting 1-24 hours with bilateral EEG slow wave abnormalities (bi-hemispheric migraine);
3. basilar type migraine with prolonged aura and diffuse EEG beta activity.

We will describe these 3 groups of patients in order to illustrate the interest of the different investigations. In a second part of this chapter, we will give examples of patients with epileptic status than can mimick migraine with atypical prolonged aura and will demonstrate how to differentiate these two types of attacks.

A proposal for an electro-clinical classification of migraine with atypical prolonged aura

Prolonged migraine aura lasting 1-24 hours with unilateral EEG slow wave abnormalities in children (Parain *et al.*, 2007)

Research into the pathophysiology of human migraine aura has been hampered by the episodic nature, short duration, and unpredictable onset of migraine attacks. Several techniques have been employed, with variable success, to evaluate the relationships and the relative importance of neuronal *versus* vascular factors associated with aura (see Chapter 1).

The migraine aura includes a variety of neurological symptoms that appear gradually before or during the development of a migraine headache. The typical aura usually lasts from 5 to 60 minutes (Headache Classification Subcommittee of the IHS, 2004), during which the EEG remains normal (Lauritzen *et al.*, 1981). The current neurogenic theory maintains that the aura is caused by a cortical spreading depression (CSD) (Lauritzen, 1994). The most direct evidence of CSD in visual aura has been obtained by magnetoencephalography (Bowyer *et al.*, 2001). The neuronal depolarisation causes slow changes in direct current magnetic field potentials in patchy areas of the corresponding occipital cortex. Olesen *et al.* (1990) were the first to study cerebral blood flow during the attack of migraine with aura. They used intra-arterial ^{133}Xe blood techniques to investigate the hemodynamic changes that occurred during aura-like symptoms induced by carotid angiography. They reported a succession of hypo and hyperperfusion predominantly in the posterior part of the brain and these modifications usually last less than 8 hours.

The SPECT technique has been used in a small series of patients (Andersen *et al.*, 1988). In most reported cases of MWA, hypoperfusion occurred during the attack. More recently, PET and BOLD functional MRI have provided the possibility of imaging the typical visual aura in migraine (Woods *et al.*, 1994; Hadjikhani *et al.*, 2001). However, these techniques do not directly record CSD. Transcranial Doppler (TCD) has also been used to investigate hemodynamic changes during MWA with controversial results (Zanette *et al.*, 1991; De Benedittis *et al.*, 1999).

In SHM, the duration of the aura is between 5 minutes and 24 hours. This type of migraine is recognized by the ICHD-II if aura includes some unilateral weakness (Headache Classification Subcommittee of the IHS, 2004). Some patients have the same duration of aura but with no weakness and are often classified as having migraine with typical aura (MWTA), even if the criteria of duration of aura is not fulfilled. In these 2 types of patients, when the duration of aura is more than 1 hour (duration criteria of MWA) but less than 24 hours (all the patients have a normal clinical status after a night sleep), abnormal focal slow waves by EEG have been reported (Sand, 1991), but the spatial and temporal distribution is not well known. Their relationships with vascular events have not yet been investigated.

The patients with clinical manifestations of this type of aura (unilateral visual disturbances, hemparesthesia, hemiparesia or aphasia) are usually admitted to the Pediatric Emergency Unit. Several investigations (EEG, TCD and SPECT) are sometimes performed to confirm the migraine type of neuro-vascular dysfunction. In this study, we report the retrospective analysis of these techniques in a group of these types of children.

Patients and methods

Between 1998 and 2004, 25 children (14 males and 11 females), from 8 to 15 years of age (mean 11 ± 2.4) were admitted to the Pediatric Emergency Unit for migraine aura with a duration between 1 and 24 hours, with or without unilateral weakness. Adequate functional investigation data for this retrospective analysis were available for only 11 of the 25 children who were admitted. For others, only clinical data have been reported. None of the patients, in this analysis reported a previous medical history of familial hemiplegic migraine or epilepsy. All had a normal brain CT-scan.

On the day of admission (D1), each patient had EEG, TCD and brain SPECT, and the same investigations were repeated on the following day (D2). The migrainous hemisphere (MH) and the non MH were defined according to the topography of neurological symptoms and the location of EEG abnormalities. The EEGs were recorded by 21 channels according to the 10-20 system. The TCD was performed with a 2 MHz probe. Mean velocities (MV) and pulsatility index were measured bilaterally on the middle cerebral arteries (MCA). The pulsatility index was calculated as the ratio: peak systolic velocity – end diastolic velocity/mean velocities and is considered as a measure of distal vascular resistance. The Wilcoxon test was used to compare MV and pulsatility index on MCA on the MH and non MH. After injection of ethyl-cysteinate dimer (bicisate) (n = 10) or hexa-methyl-propylene-amone-Oxime (exametazzime) (n = 1), the SPECT was performed on a dual headed camera (DST-XL, GEMS). Projections were reconstructed using filtered back projection (Gaussien filter: = 2.8). Five cerebral regions of interest (ROI) (calcarine, middle occipital, superior occipital, middle temporal and frontal) were drawn on each hemisphere by using the Talairach atlas. The perfusion index was calculated for each ROI as the ratio of cortical perfusion/cerebellum perfusion. Analysis of variance was used to compare perfusion index between the MH and non MH on D1 and on D2.

Results

Of the 11 patients, who underwent the above investigations, 9 had visual symptoms, 4 had hemiparesis with numbness on the same side, 3 had aphasia and 5 a decreased level of consciousness. For the 14 other patients, 11 had visual symptoms, 4 had hemiparesis with homolateral numbness, 2 aphasia and 5 a decreased level of consciousness. The minimal duration of the aura was 5 hours. The maximal duration of the aura was sometimes difficult to determine, but, after a night's sleep, all the patients felt very well and had a normal clinical status. All patients had migraine headache during the attack. In these 25 patients, 12 patients fulfilled the criteria of MWTA (with at least 2 attacks), 6 patients fulfilled the criteria of SHM. For 4 patients, it was the first attack of MWA, but they previously had experienced attacks of migraine without aura.

On D1 *(Fig. 1a)*, the TCDs of all patients showed a decrease of MV on MCA in the MH (mean 50 cm/s; SD 8.5), compared with the non MH (mean 61 cm/s; SD 12.7; $p = 0.04$). In addition, the pulsatility index on the MH (mean 1.19) was increased as compared with the non-MH (mean 0.92; $p = 0.002$). On D2 *(Fig. 1b)*, the increase of MV on the MCA in the MH was not considered significant.

The EEGs of 2 patients were performed within 2-3 hours of the beginning of aura (hemiparesia for one and visual symptoms associated with drowsiness for the other), and the results were normal. These normal EEGs were associated with a slowing on MCA and diffuse or focal hypoperfusion on MH *(Fig. 2a and 2c)*. The EEGs of the remaining 9 patients, which were performed after 3 hours on D1, were abnormal and showed unilateral slow-wave abnormalities on MH, temporo-occipital for 8 patients *(Fig. 3a)*, diffuse for 1 patient *(Fig. 4a)*, and associated with a hypoperfusion in the same area *(Fig. 3c and 4c)*. On D2, the EEGs of all patients showed rhythmic slow-wave abnormalities only on the occipital area of MH with a good reactivity at the opening of the eyes *(Fig. 2, 3, 4b)*. The MH of each patient was well defined by a concordance between the topography, the type of neurological symptoms and the lateralization of EEG abnormalities.

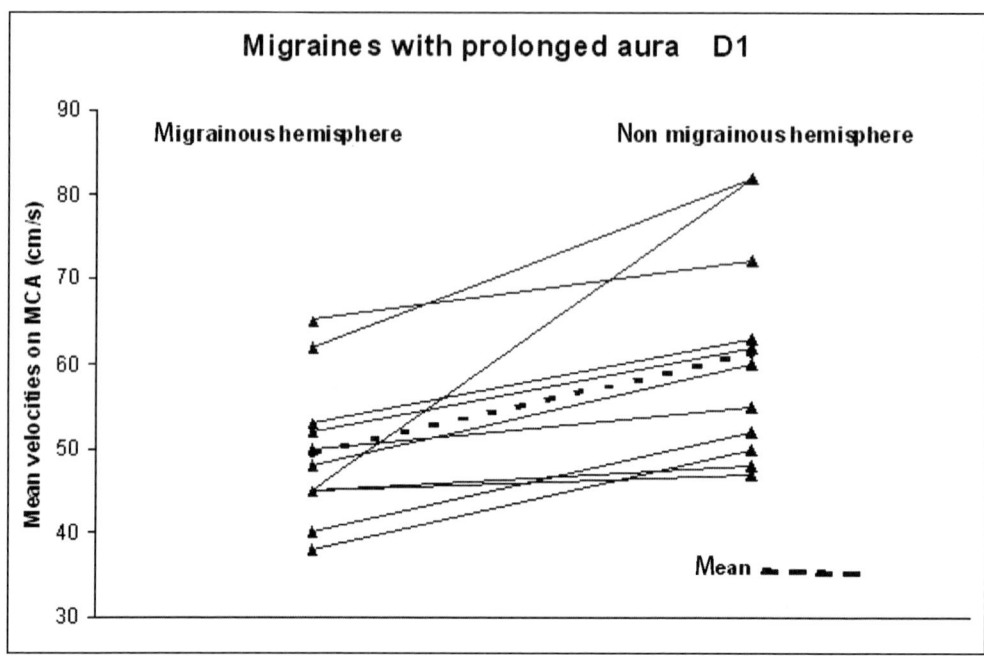

Figure 1a. TCD at D1 (MV on MCA).

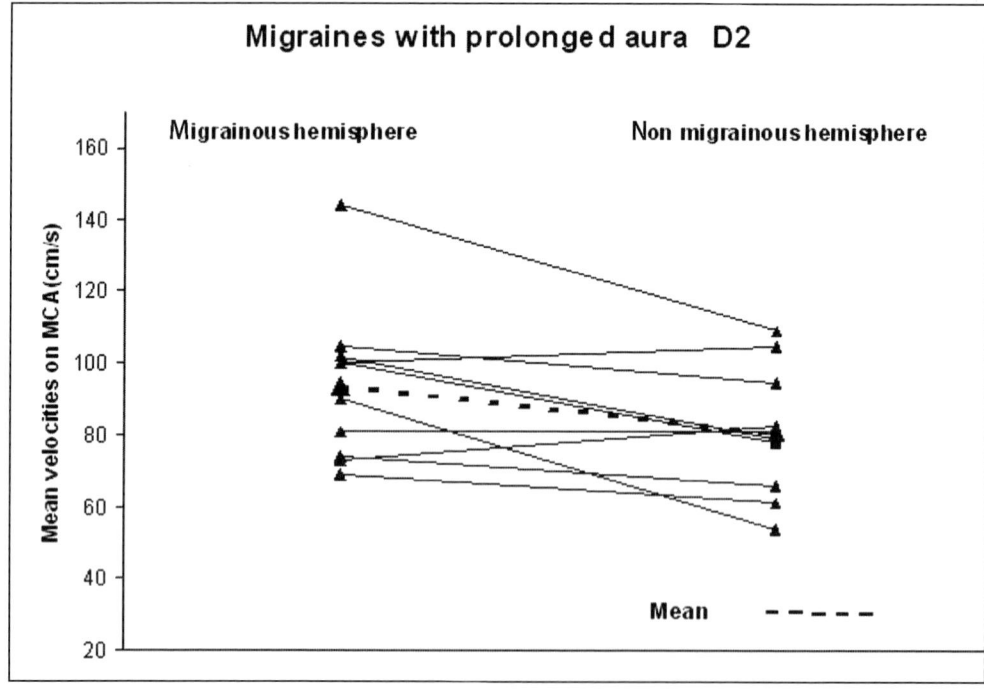

Figure 1b. TCD at D2 (MV on MCA).

Differential diagnosis between epilepsy and particular forms of migraine

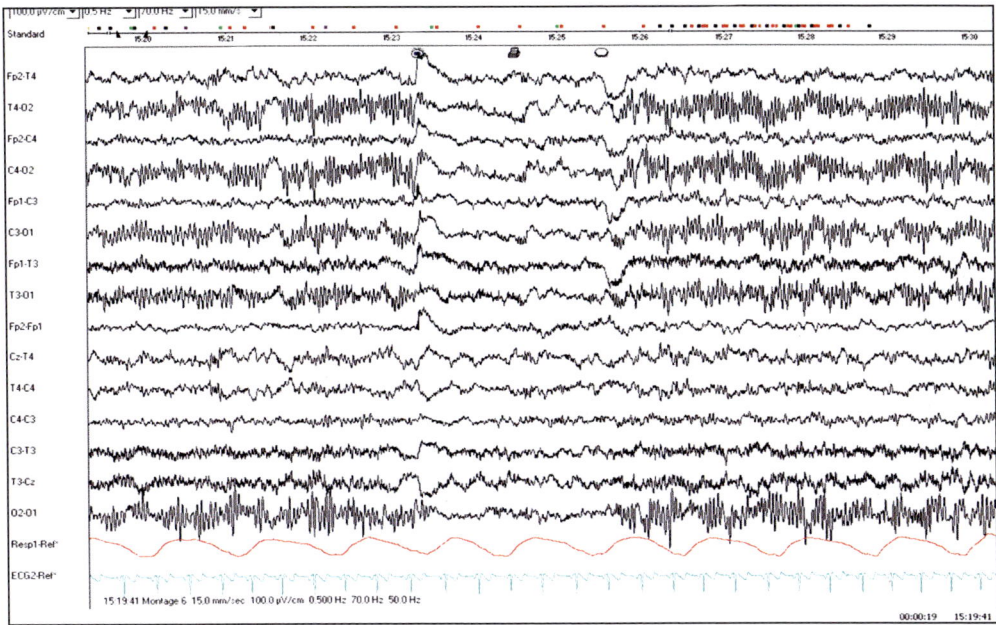

Figure 2a. Patient with right hemiparesis and headache: the EEG was preformed 3 hours after the beginning of aura (D1) and was normal. In the same time, TCD showed a decrease MV on left MCA (45 cm/s) compared to the right side (80 cm/s).

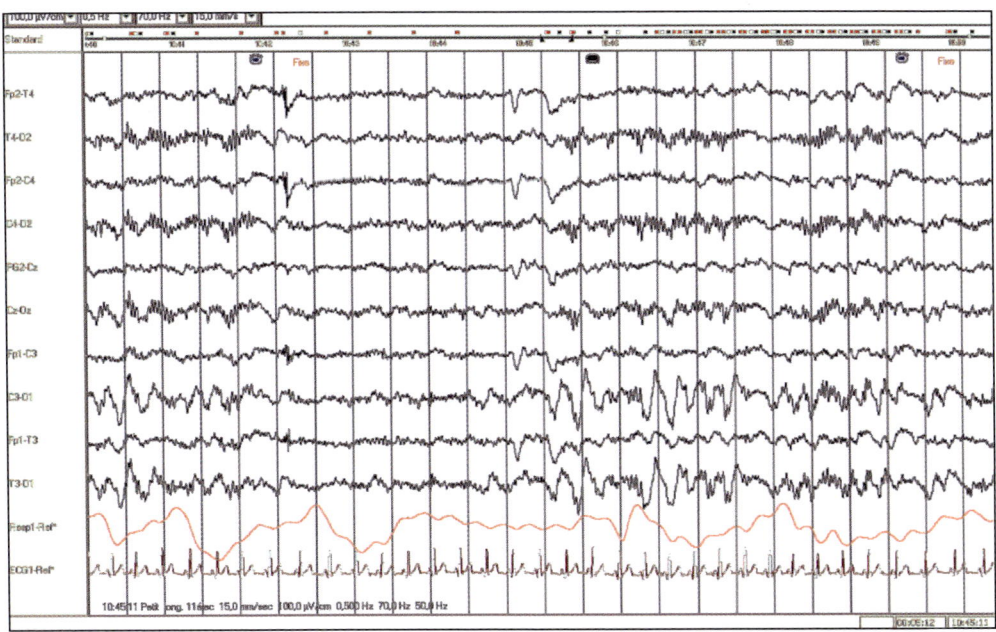

Figure 2b. The same patient at D2 with high amplitude EEG slow waves abnormalities in the left occipital area.

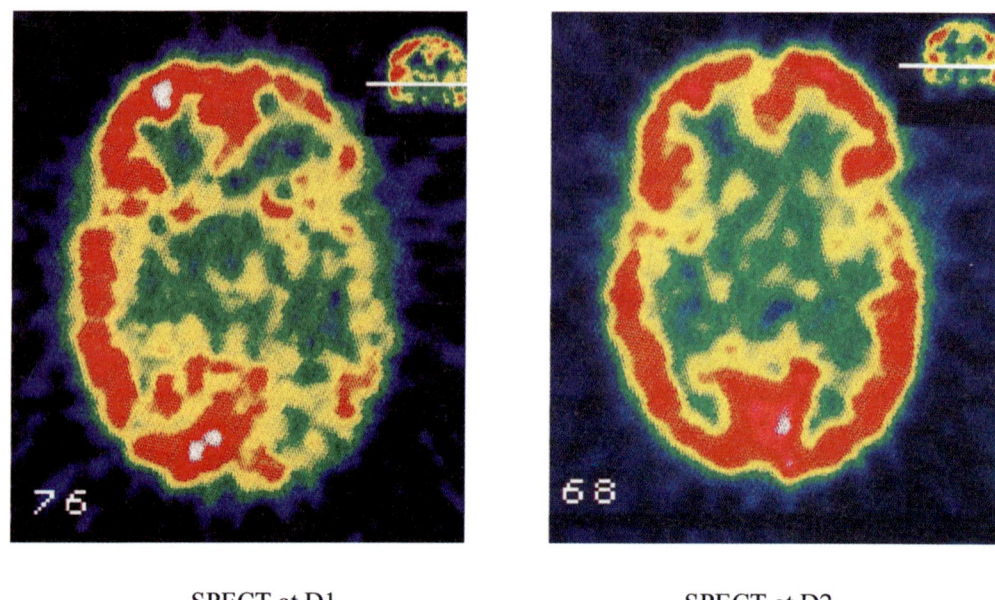

SPECT at D1   SPECT at D2

Figure 2c. At D1, the SPECT, performed 4 hours after the beginning of aura, showed 20% diffuse left hypoperfusion and at D2, the SPECT showed 14% hyperperfusion in the left occipito-temporal.

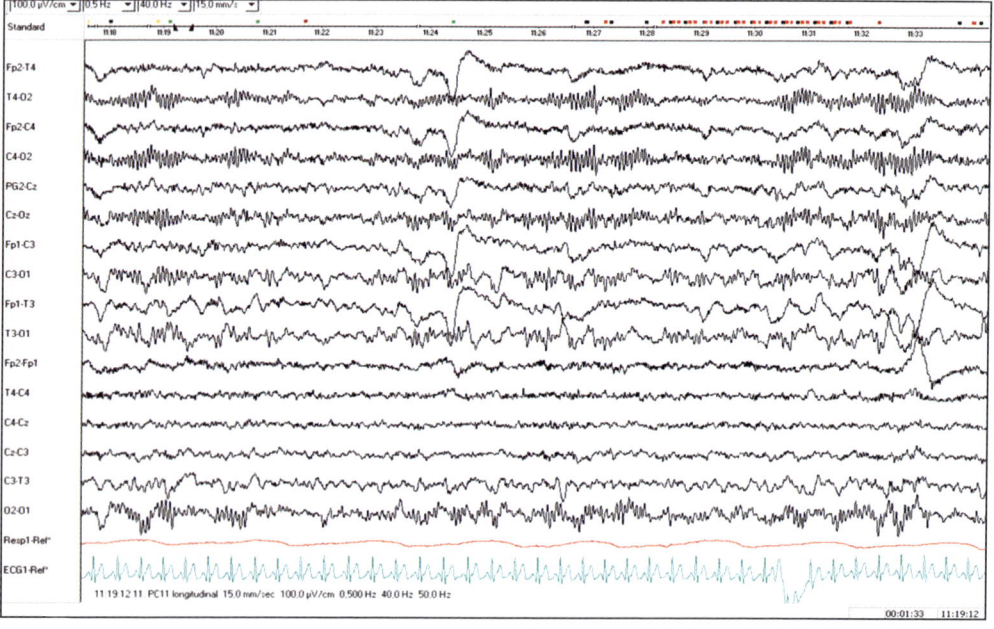

Figure 3a. Another patient with aphasia and headache at D1. The EEG were performed at 7 hours with left tempo-occipital slow waves abnormalities.

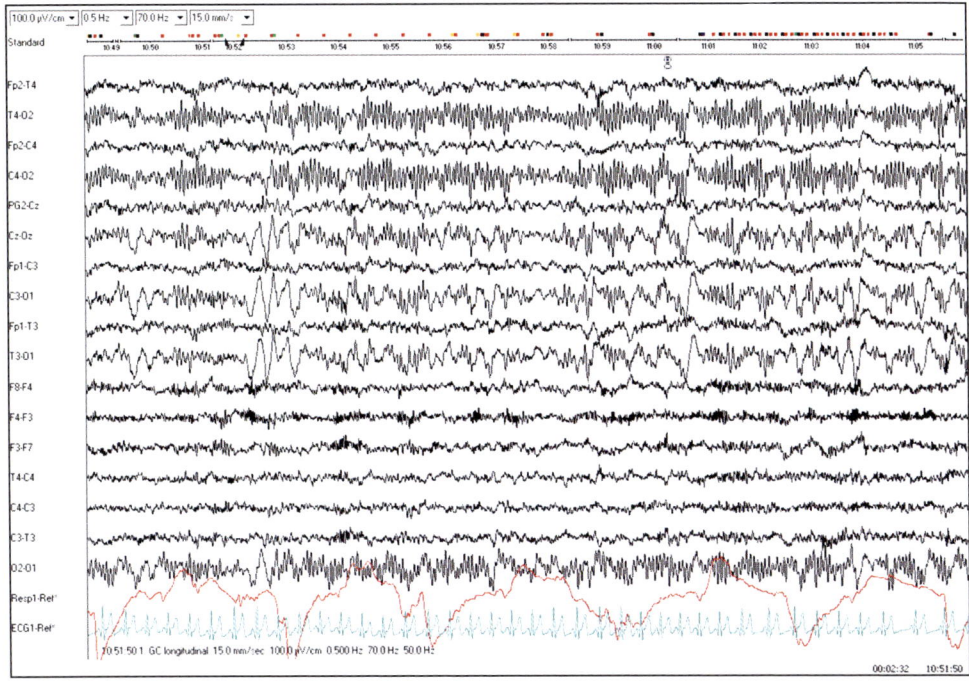

Figure 3b. The same patient at D2: strictly left occipital EEG slow waves abnormalities.

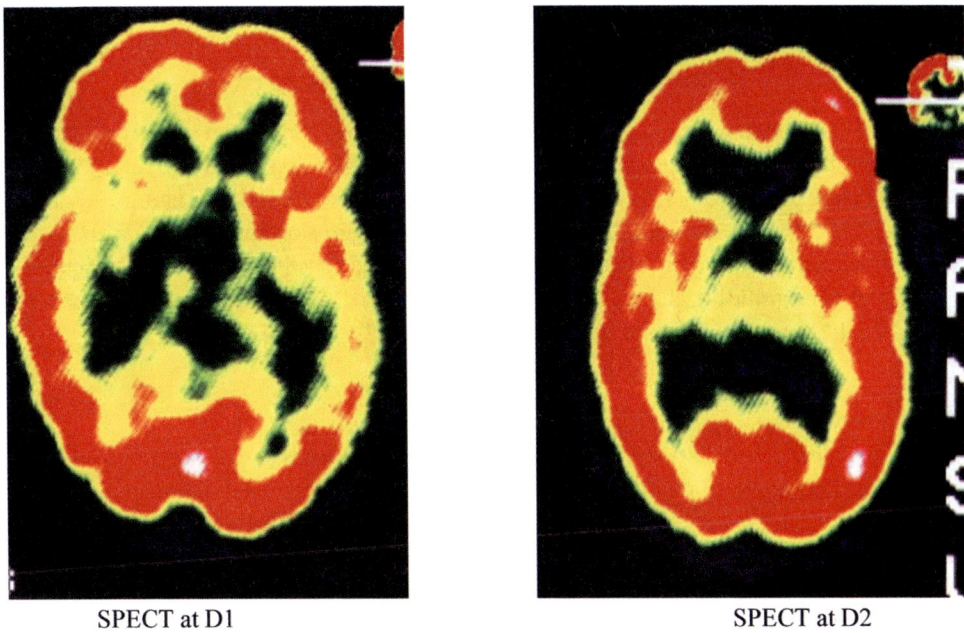

SPECT at D1 　　　　　　　　　　　　　　SPECT at D2

Figure 3c. The same patient with left temporal hyperpufusion at SPECT perfommed at 12 hours at D1. The SPECT at D2 showed an hyperperfusion on the left occipito-temporal area.

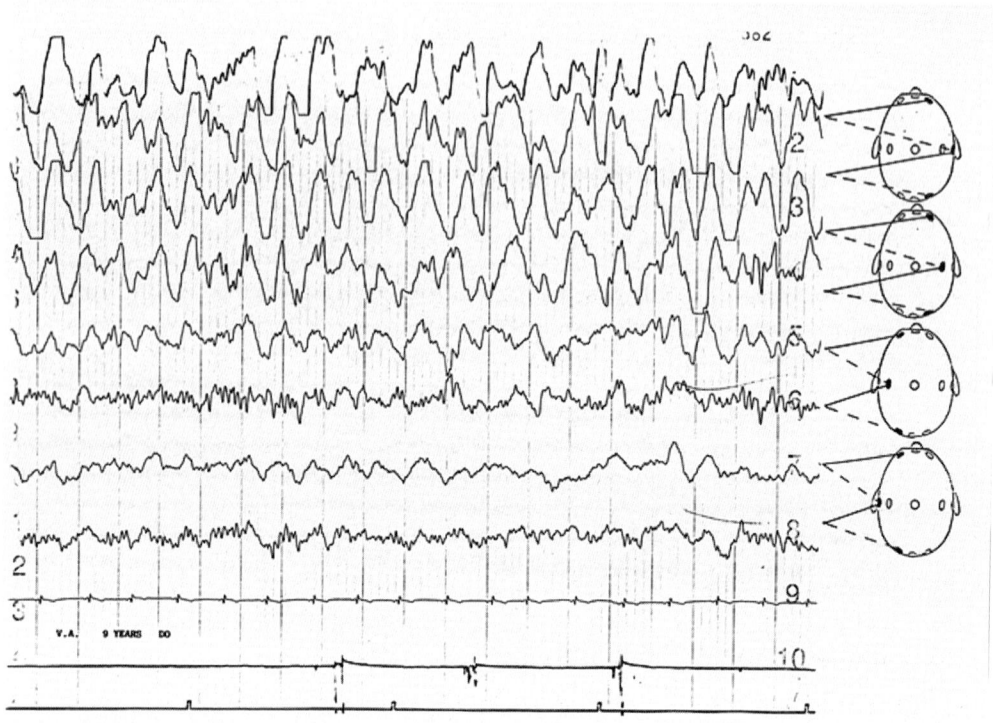

Figure 4a. Patient at D1 with right high amplitude diffuse EEG slow waves abnormalities.

On D1, the SPECT of each patient showed a hypoperfusion in several ROI on the MH as compared with the non MH. The mean perfusion index of each of the 4 occipital and temporal ROI of the MH significantly decreased (- 13% to - 15%; $0.0014 < p < 0.0076$) on D1 and significantly increased (+ 6%; $0.0021 < p < 0.01$) on D2. A comparison of the perfusion index on DI with those of the D2 revealed a significant change of these four ROI (+ 15 to + 19%; $0.0001 < p < 0.0064$) on the MH, but no significant change in any ROI on the non MH. No significant changes were observed in the perfusion index of the bilateral frontal ROI.

Discussion

The time of appearance of EEG abnormalities in migrainous aura has to date remained unknown. However, the EEG has been reported to remain normal during the usual duration aura of MWTA (5-60 minutes) (Lauritzen et al., 1981). In two of our patients, recorded during the first 3 hours, EEGs were normal. When the EEGs were recorded after 3 hours on D1, slow-wave abnormalities were always observed on the MH, either temporo-occipital or diffuse. Therefore, this could suggest that the EEG abnormalities appear between 1 and 3 hours after the beginning of aura. On D2, the slow-wave abnormalities were only occipital in the same hemisphere, which is associated with a normal clinical status.

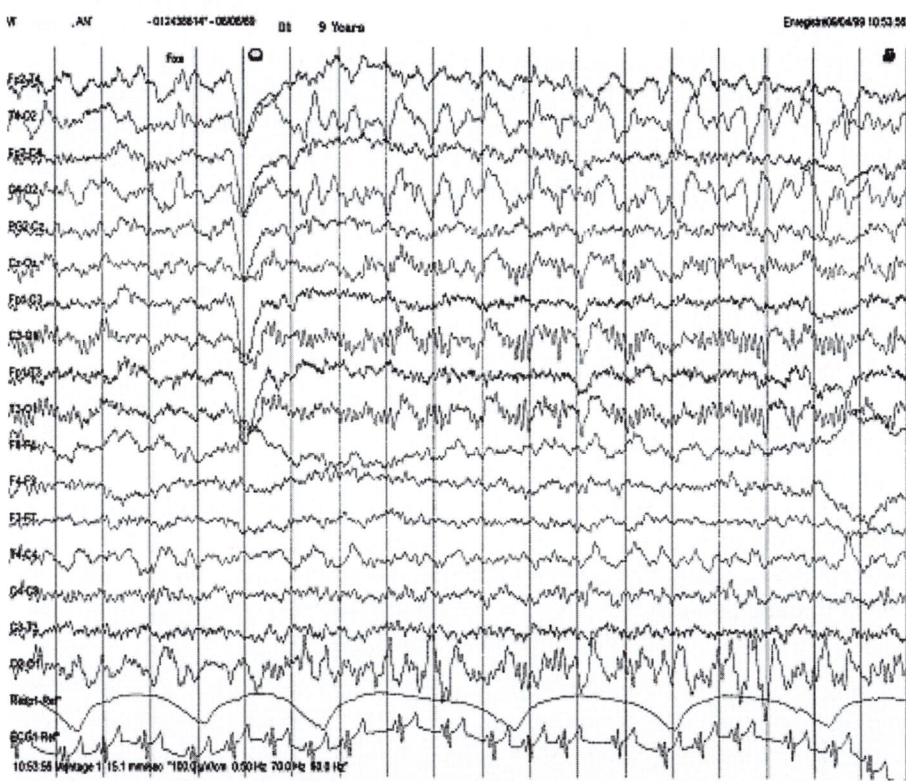

Figure 4b. Same patient at D2: right occipital EEG slow waves.

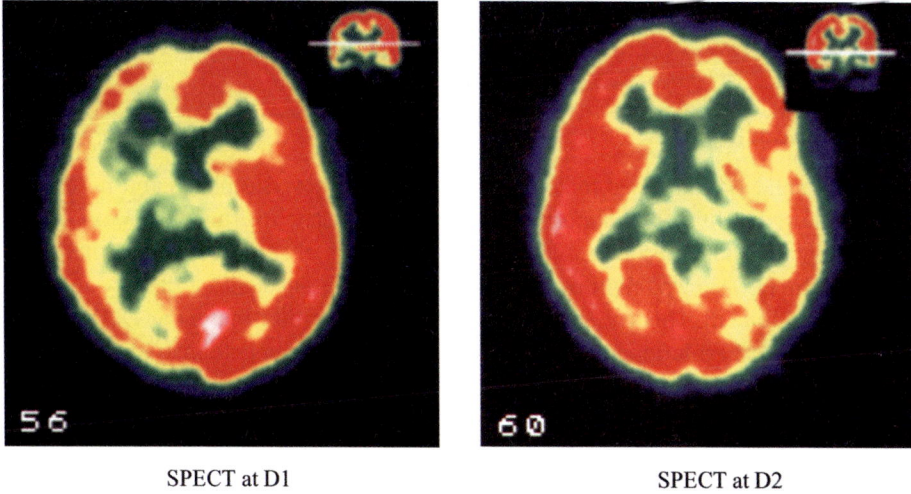

SPECT at D1   SPECT at D2

Figure 4c. The SPECT at D1 showed a diffuse right hypoperfusion and the SPECT at D2 showed a diffuse hyperperfusion on the same hemisphere.

In rats, CSD can be observed by application of potassium chloride on the cerebral cortex. The electrocorticogram initially records an electrical silence, followed, some minutes later, by abnormal slow waves before complete restoration. Several waves of depressed neuronal activity were propagated across the brain cortex at 2 to 3 mm/min and associated with a reduction in cerebral blood flow. At the beginning of human aura, the electrical volume of CSD conduction is too small to evoke EEG abnormalities, but sufficiently large to be detected by magnetoencephalography and to cause neurological symptoms. The slow wave abnormalities appear after several hours, probably due to the increase in the area of electrical volume of CSD conduction. These slow waves are probably the direct expression of the CSD restoration phase. The localization of EEG abnormalities on the D2 in the occipital lobe of the migrainous hemisphere in each patient could be due to a particular predisposition of this brain area to CSD.

According to the literature and our data, the hypoperfusion seems to appear very early in aura. This hypoperfusion is below the threshold of ischemia and is not severe enough to be the cause of clinical symptoms. It is classically admitted that the hypoperfusion in aura is secondary to CSD although some contradictory data have been previously reported (Goadsby, 2005). For one of our patients, a diffuse unilateral hypoperfusion was associated with a controlateral hemiparesis and a normal EEG during the first hours of aura. The areas of spreading depression were probably too limited to cause EEG abnormalities and diffuse unilateral hypoperfusion. Some brainstem nucleus may play a role in triggering the hypoperfusion.

The sequence of EEG and TCD abnormalities in migraine aura can be useful as a diagnostic tool. The succession of unilateral diffuse or temporo-occipital EEG slow waves abnormalities associated with a slowing of MV on homolateral MCA at D1, follows at D2 by a normal clinical status and occipital slow waves on the same side which confirms the diagnosis of migraine, if the clinical symptoms are concordant with this diagnosis. SPECT is not required if the TCD data are significant. In our experience, if at D2, the clinical status is not completely normal and the EEG abnormalities are not strictly occipital, the diagnosis of familial hemiplegic migraine remains debatable.

Addendum

A 12 year old child was admitted for impaired of consciousness, sleepiness and headache. The EEG at D1 showed right frontal abnormalities *(Fig. 5a)* associated with slow MV on right MCA and right frontal hypoperfusion at SPECT *(Fig. 5b)*. The patient's status was normal after one night. At D2 the EEG showed right occipital slow waves associated with a right occipital hyperperfusion *(Fig. 5c and d)*. This patient had an atypical localization of aura at DI in the frontal area, but with typical evolution at D2. This observation is a further demonstration that the EEG at D2, in this type of unilateral aura, always shows occipital slow waves abnormalities even if the neurovascular dysfunction is located on frontal area at D1.

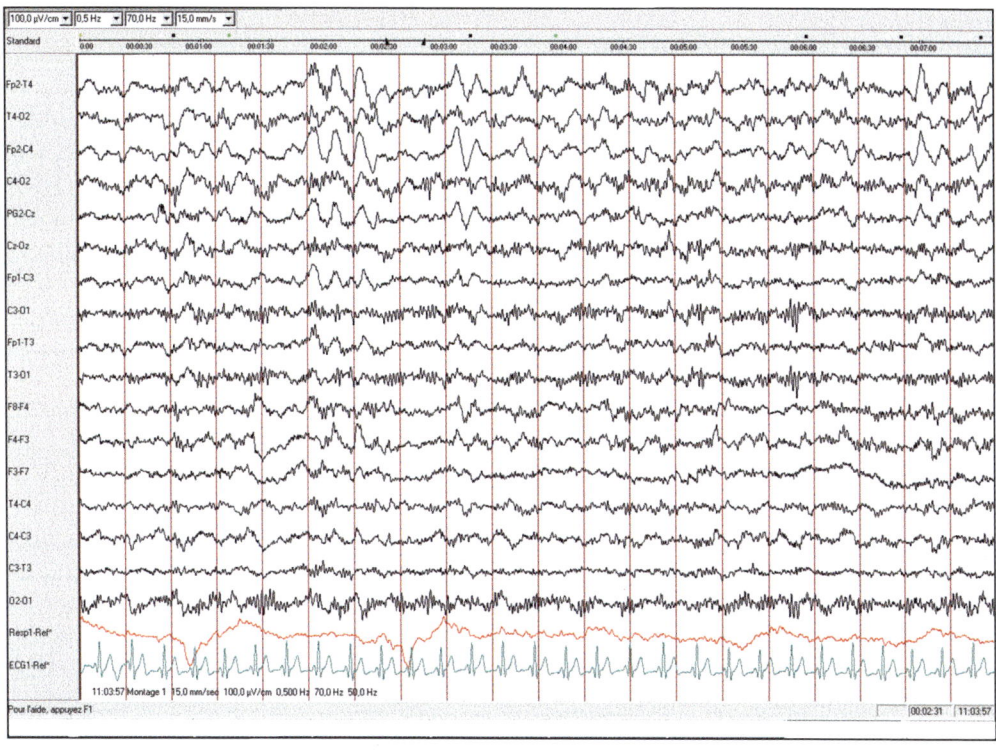

Figure 5a. Patient at D1 with right frontal slow waves abnormalities.

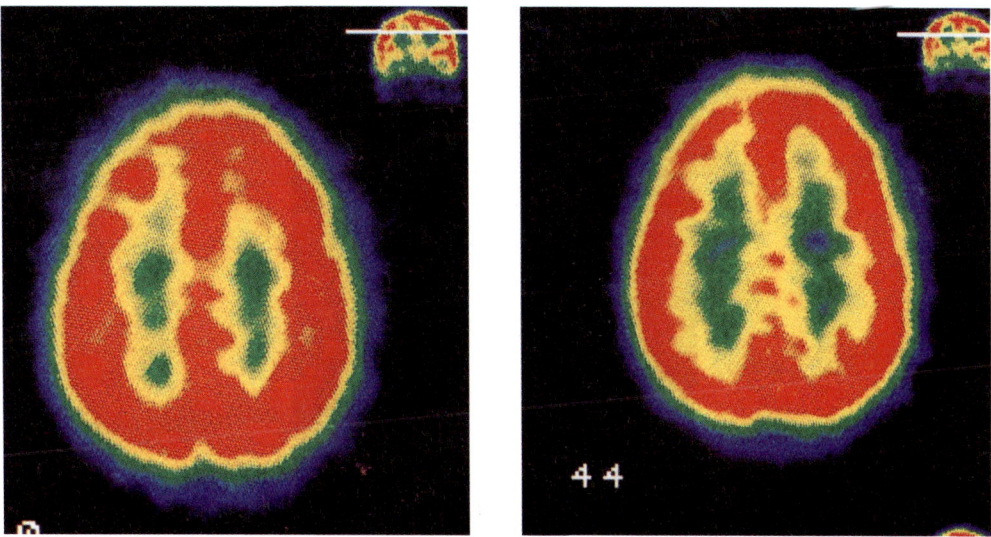

Figure 5b. SPECT showed right frontal hypoperfusion at D1.

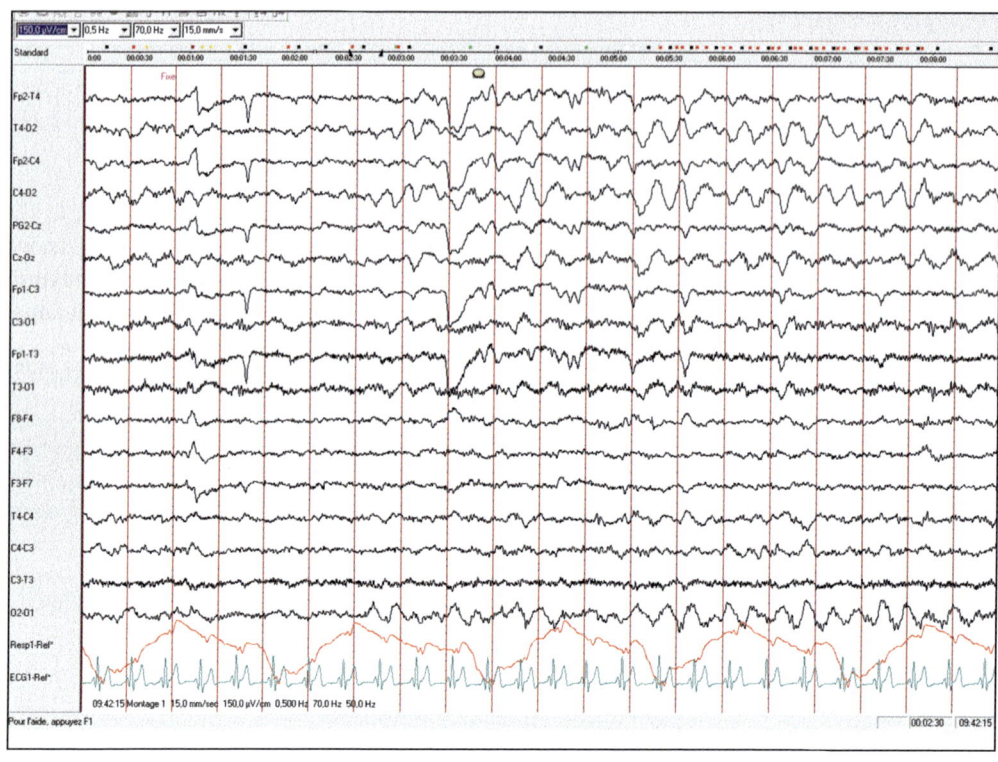

Figure 5c. Same patient at D2: right occipital slow waves abnormalities.

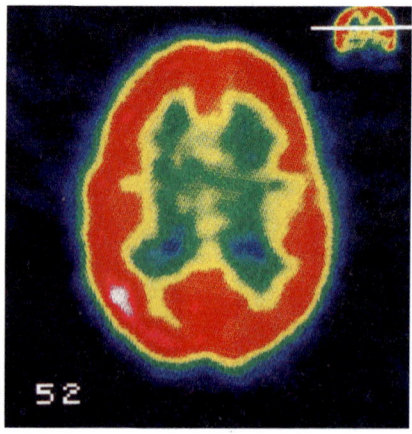

Figure 5d. Same patient with right temporo-occipital hyperperfusion at D2.

Prolonged migraine aura lasting 1-24 hours with bilateral EEG slow wave abnormalities (bi-hemispheric migraine)

We have grouped, in this section, patients with the same dysfunction as that previously mentioned, but on both hemispheres. Some of these patients may be classified as ACM described by Gascon and Barlow (1970) but not all of these patients were confused. According to ICHD-II, these patients should have been classified as having a bi-hemispheric form of BTM. However, we prefer the term bi-hemispheric migraine (BHM) because, as we will demonstrate, brainstem symptoms are limited and there is a major involvement of MCA circulation in this type of migraine.

The spatial and temporal distribution of EEG abnormalities in these patients will be discussed later. To date, their relationships to vascular events have not been investigated. These patients are usually admitted to the Pediatric Emergency Unit. Several investigations (CT scan, EEG, TCD) are sometimes performed to confirm a migraine type neuro-vascular dysfunction. In this study, we report the retrospective analysis of clinical data and the results of these techniques in this pediatric population.

Patients and methods

Between 1999 and 2004, 7 children (4 males and 3 females), aged 8 to 14 years (mean 11 ± 1.8) were admitted to the Pediatric Emergency Unit for BHM with a duration of aura between 1 and 24 hours. None of the patients, in this analysis, had a previous medical history of FHM or epilepsy. All had a normal brain CT-scan.

On the day of admission (D1), each patient had EEG, TCD and the same tests were repeated on the following day (D2) and on D30 (baseline) for the TCD. The EEGs were recorded by 21 channels according to the 10-20 system. The TCD was performed with a 2 MHz probe. MV and pulsatility index were measured bilaterally on the MCA. The Wilcoxon test was used to compare MV and pulsatility index on the both MCA between D1 and D30 and then between D2 and D30.

Results

The patients had at least 2 reversible symptoms required for MWA diagnostic criteria. Three had visual symptoms, 6 had decreased level of consciousness, 4 had speech disorders, 2 had bilateral paresthesia and 3 had vertigo. Additional symptoms, not included in diagnostic criteria of MWA, were observed as agitation (3 patients), confusion (4 patients). One patient had BHM after minor head trauma. The minimal duration of the aura was 4 hours. The maximal duration of the aura was sometimes difficult to determine, but, after a night's sleep, all the patients felt very well and had a normal clinical status. All patients had migraine headache during the attack. In these 7 patients, 3 patients had at least 2 attacks of BHM. For 4 patients, it was their first attack of BHM, but they had previously experienced several attacks of migraine without aura.

On D1, the TCDs of all patients showed a decrease of MV of the right MCA (mean 56 cm/s; SD 15), compared with baseline (mean 77 cm/s; SD 15; $p = 0.02$) and on the left MCA (mean 51 cm/s; SD 13), compared with baseline (mean 70 cm/s; SD 14; $p = 0.02$) *(Fig. 6)*. In addition, the

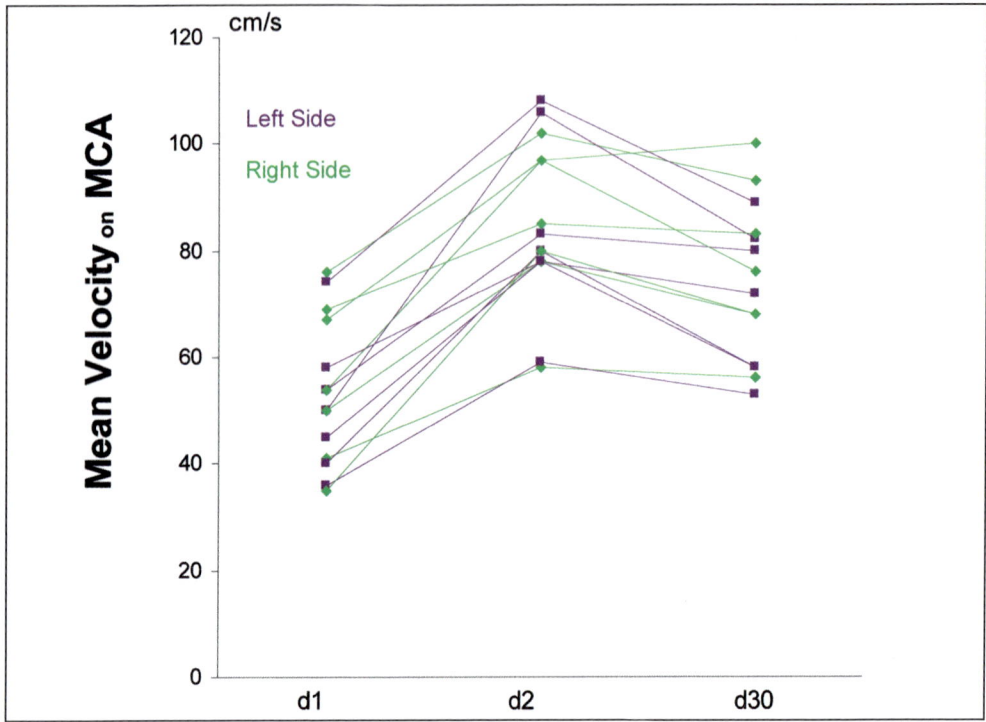

Figure 6. TCD on the both right and left MCA of the 7 patients with BHM: MV at D1, D2 and D30 (baseline).

pulsatility index was increased on the right MCA (mean 1.22) as compared with baseline (mean 0.91; p = 0.004) and on left MCA (mean 1.14) compared baseline (mean: 0.86; p = 0.01) *(Fig. 1)*. On D2, the increase on the left MCA (mean 84 cm/s) was considered significant compared to the baseline (p = 0.02) but the increase in MV of the right MCA was not significant.

The EEGs of all the patients were performed within 4-8 hours from the beginning of aura on D1. They showed either diffuse slow-wave abnormalities *(Fig. 7a)* in 4 patients with mainly confusion, agitation, decreased level of consciousness, either bitemporo-occipital slow-waves *(Fig. 8a)* for 3 patients with mainly visual symptoms. On D2, the EEGs of all patients only showed slow-wave abnormalities on both occipital areas with a good reactivity at the opening of the eyes *(Fig. 7 and 8b)*.

Discussion

There is a clear similarity between the EEG and TCD abnormalities in the patients reported in our previous study (Parain *et al.*, 2007) where the abnormalities were unilateral and in patients with BHM where the abnormalities were bilateral. In both groups of patients, the sequence was the same: on D1, diffuse or temporo-occipital EEG slow waves were associated with a decrease of mean velocities on MCA. On D2, the EEG slow waves abnormalities were only on the occipital area associated with a slight increase of mean velocities on MCA and a normal clinical status. As

Differential diagnosis between epilepsy and particular forms of migraine

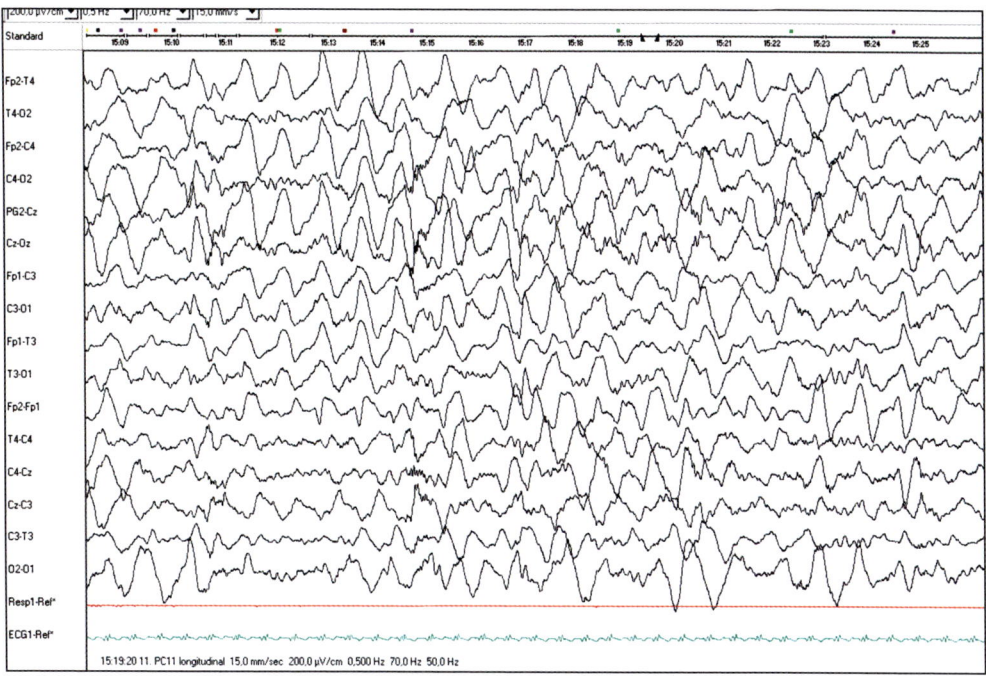

Figure 7a. Patient with BHM at D1: high amplitude diffuses slow waves abnormalities.

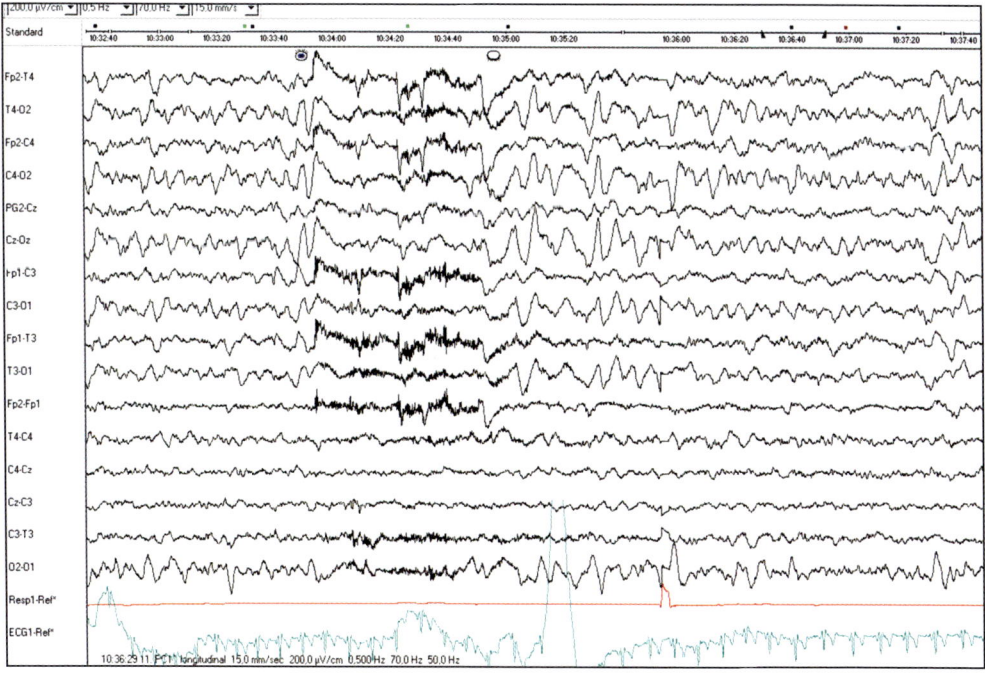

Figure 7b. Same patient at D2: bi-occipital slow waves, reacting at the opening of the eyes.

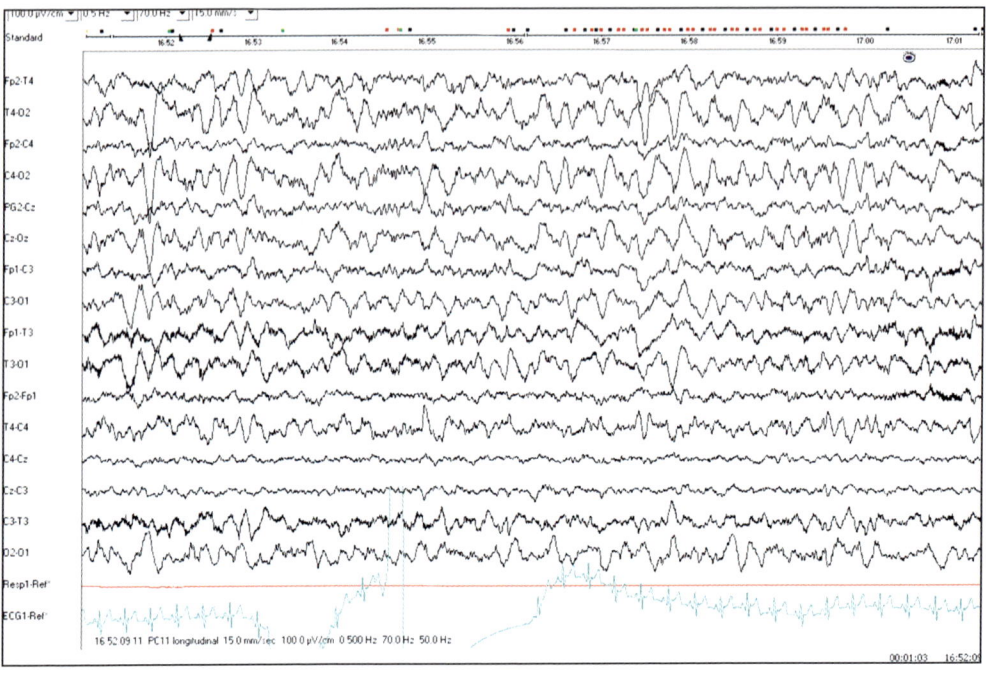

Figure 8a. EEG of another patient with BHM and bi-occipito-temporal slow waves on D1.

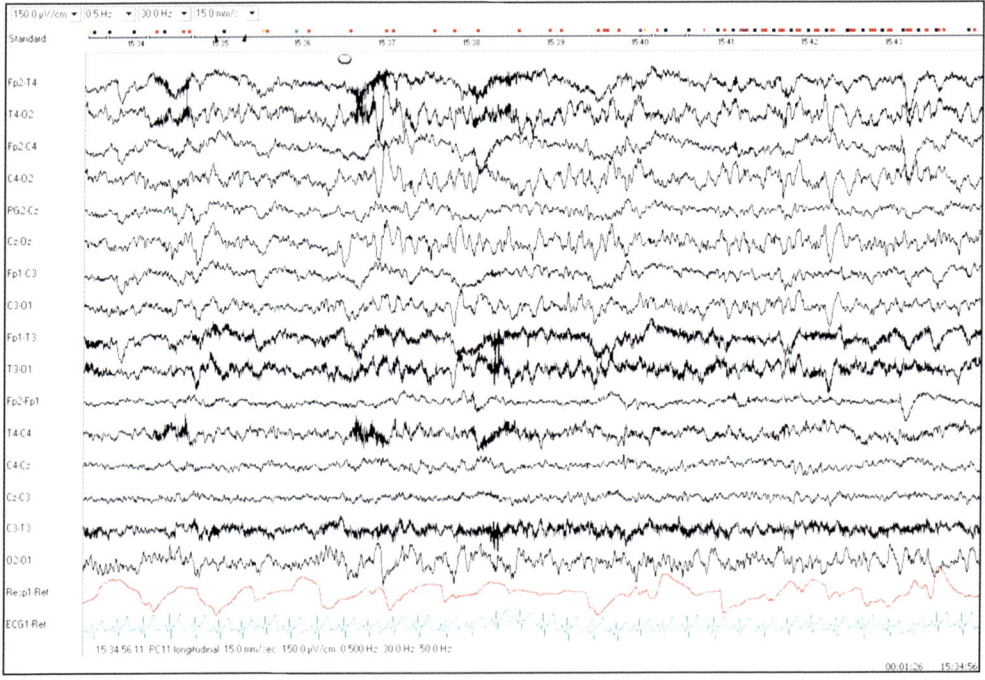

Figure 8b. Same patient: bioccipital slow waves, blocking at the open eyes.

shown by the TCD abnormalities, the involvement of MCA territory was evident in these patients with BHM. Only 2 patients had visual disturbances and 2 with vertigo. None had other brainstem symptoms. The 4 patients with diffuse EEG slow waves at DI in this study are in agreement with the diagnosis of ACM. In 3 patients with temporo-occipital EEG, slow waves were similar to the same patients as reported by Lapkin *et al.* (1977) with both visual and brainstem symptom. As in our previous study (Parain *et al.*, 2007), the EEG slow wave abnormalities probably need several hours after the beginning of aura to appear and are the direct expression of the restoration phase of CSD. The localization of these slow waves on D2 in both occipital lobes in each patient is perhaps due to a particular predisposition of this brain area to CSD. EEG and TCD remain useful tools to diagnose migraine aura lasting 1-24 hours and to localize the main site of dysfunction.

Basilar type migraine with prolonged aura and diffuse EEG beta activity (Parain and Samson-Dollfus, 1984)

We have grouped, in this section, patients with symptoms compatible with BTM according to ICHD-II but with prolonged aura and diffuse fast rhythms on EEG. Lapkin *et al.* (1977) reported bilateral occipital slow waves abnormalities at D2 in patients with basilar migraine, but all patients primarily had visual disturbances and probably had BHM with typical EEG at D2. Diffuse EEG beta activity in BTM with prolonged aura has previously been reported by Parain and Samson-Dollfus (1984) and Soriani *et al.* (1996).

Between 1979 and 1983, 9 children (6 males and 3 females) aged from 9 to 14, were hospitalized for attacks of brainstem symptomatology evoking BTM and their data have previously been reported (Parain and Samson-Dollfus, 1984). Since 1983, we have collected the data of 6 other patients with a similar clinical presentation.

Patients and method

We reported the data of 15 patients who were admitted to our Pediatric Emergency Unit since 1979 for BTM with prolonged aura (> 1 hour). They were 8 males and 7 females, aged from 8 to 15 years.

All patients had ataxia, vertigo, diplopia and headache during the attack. Four were mildly confused with a slightly impaired consciousness. Three had nausea. The duration of aura was between 12 hours and 3 days. None had agitation. Four patients had recurrent attacks of BTM with prolonged aura. All also had MWA.

EEGs were performed in each patient at D1 and each day after until normalization of the clinical status. TCD in MCA, posterior cerebral artery and basilar artery were performed in 5 patients. In all patients, drug intoxication had been ruled out by blood test.

Results

In each patient, the EEG showed a diffuse beta activity until the clinical status was normal *(Fig. 9a)*. The spectral analysis permitted a clear distinction between beta activity (narrow window) and muscle artifacts (large window) *(Fig. 9b)*. Within 2 or 3 days, the EEG was normal with occipital, reactive, alpha rhythm *(Fig. 9c)* in 2 or 3 days. No EEG slow waves abnormalities were observed in these patients. The TCD was normal in the 5 patients when performed, either on MCA or in posterior circulation.

Discussion

Patients with prolonged BTM aura and diffuse EEG beta activity are probably under-diagnosed for several reasons. EEG is rarely recorded to investigate the association of acute ataxia, diplopia ad vertigo. When the EEG is performed, drug intoxication is often the sole evoked diagnosis. There are some clinical differences between patients with prolonged BM and patients with benzodiazepine intoxication. In cases of prolonged BTM, patients are rarely in coma or with a major decrease in consciousness. The recovery may be longer in BTM. Diffuse EEG beta activity in BTM with prolonged aura may be trigger by brainstem nucleus dysfunction.

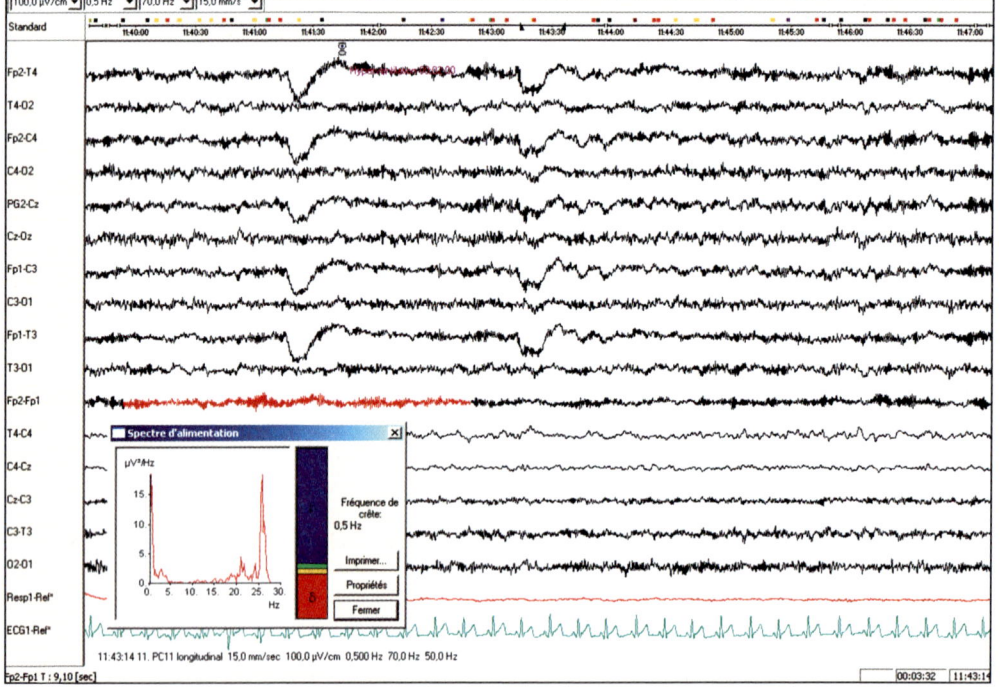

Figure 9a. Patient at D1 with BTM and brainstem symptomatology: diffuse EEG beta activity and narrow window at spectral analysis.

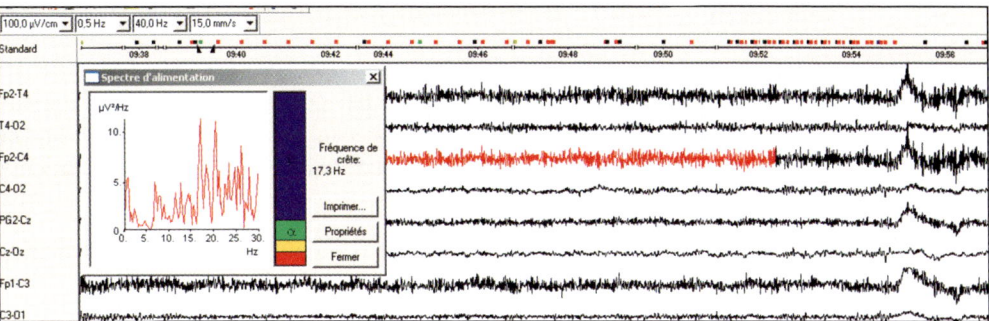

Figure 9b. Spectral analysis of muscle artifacts (large window).

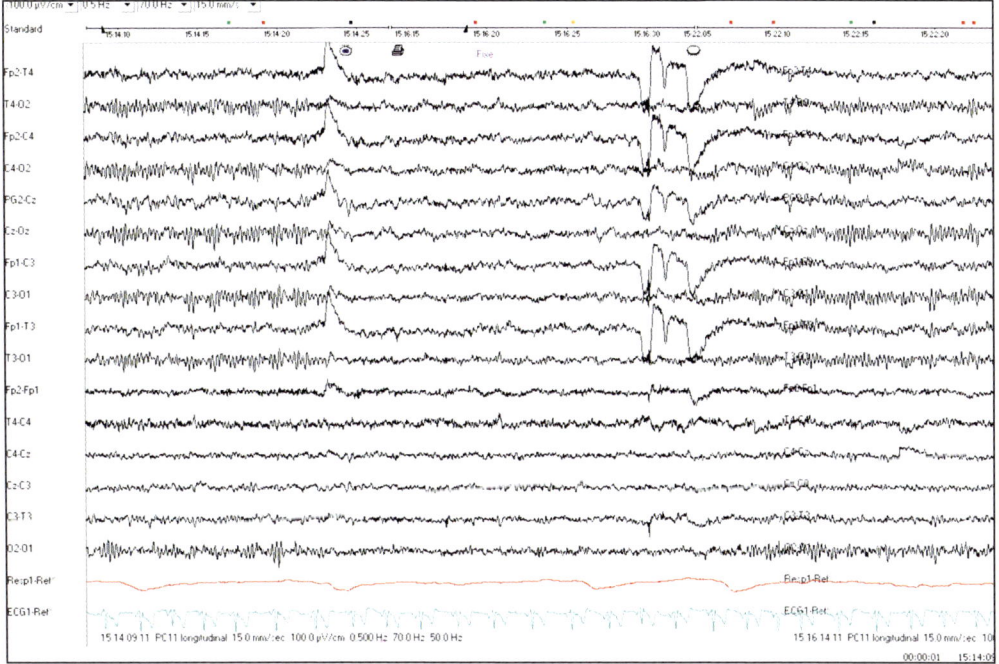

Figure 9c. Same patient at D2: normal EEG.

Beaumanoir (1993) reported short bouts of fast rhythms during the positive symptoms of a visual aura and this has been interpreted as epileptiform activity concomitant to a period of hyperexcitability. Several authors have reported other types of epileptiform activity during migraine, sometimes without aura (De Romanis *et al.*, 1993; Parisi *et al.*, 2007). In none of our patients with prolonged aura, types of epileptiform activity were recorded. Epileptic seizures may be associated with BTM in some patients and interictal occipital spikes and waves were recorded on EEG (Camfield, 1978). However, in most patients with BTM, there is no epileptic seizure and the interictal EEG is normal.

Addendum

A 15-year old girl was admitted for aphasia, sleepiness and vertigo. The EEG abnormalities at D1 were asymmetrical with predominant slow-waves on the left hemisphere during waking and sleepiness *(Fig. 10a and b)*. However, during sleep, there was an excess of beta activity on the right hemisphere *(Fig. 10b)*. At D2, the EEG showed left occipital slow waves and the patient's status was normal.

The EEG abnormalities of the patient with asymmetrical BHM and unilateral beta activity during sleep *(Fig. 3)* were probably an overlap type 2 (BHM) and type 3 (BTM) of the electro-clinical classification that we have previously proposed.

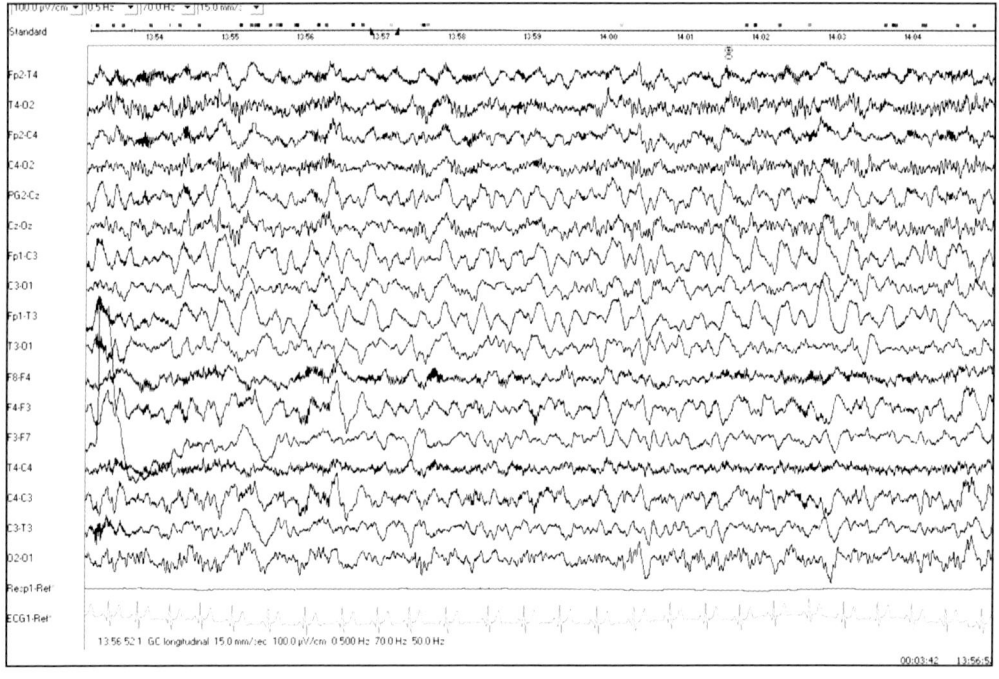

Figure 10a. Patient at D1 with a asymetrical BHM: slow waves abnormalities more marked on the left hemisphere during the wake.

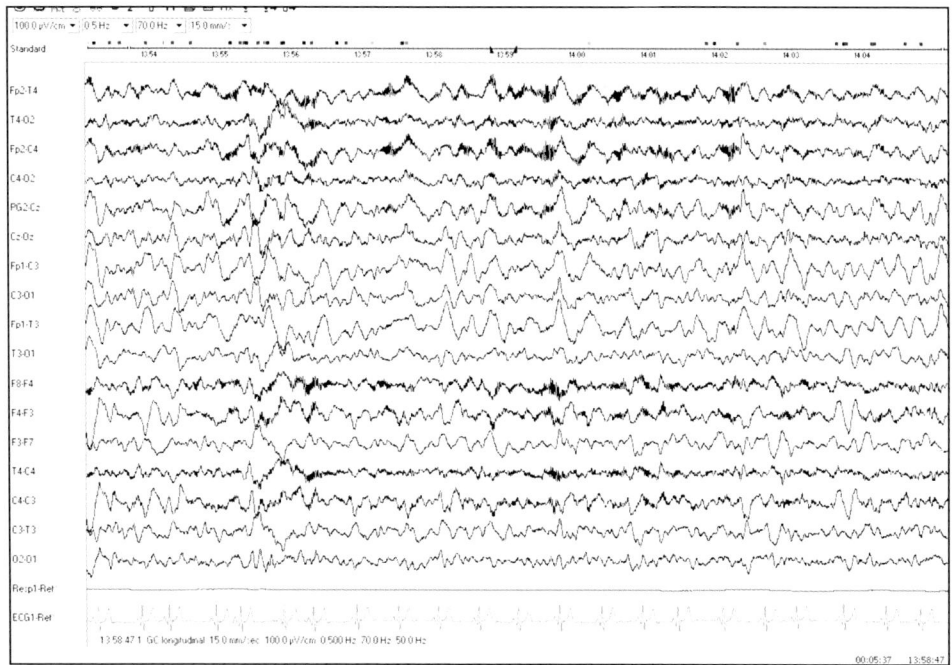

Figure 10b. Same patient at D1 during sleep: an excess of beta rhythms on the right hemisphere.

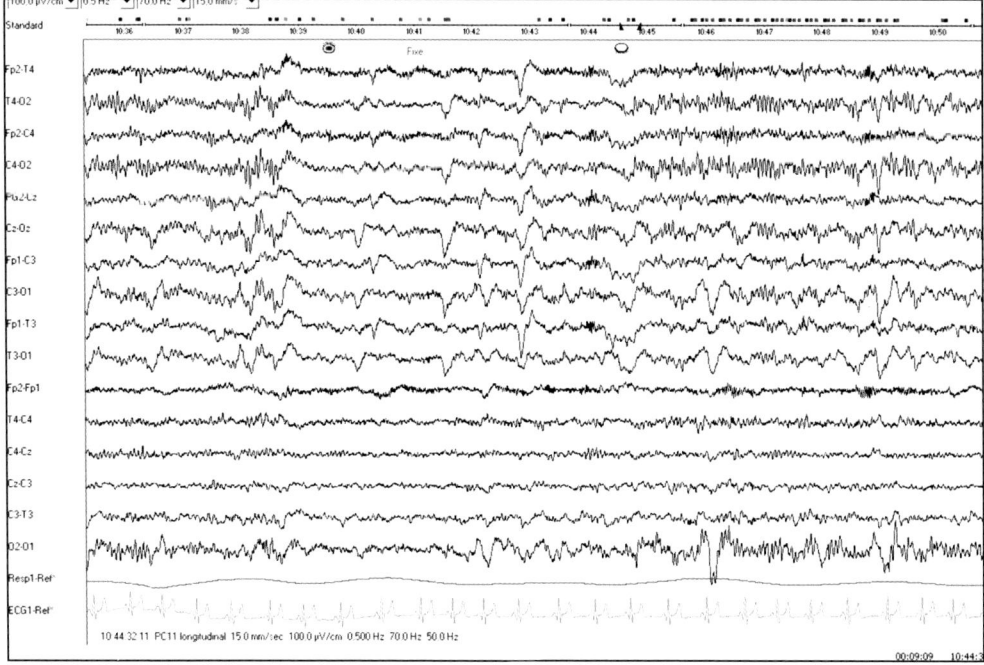

Figure 10c. Same patient at D2: left occipital reactive slow waves.

Occipital epileptic status that mimick migraine with prolonged aura

Patients with occipital status epilepticus may mimick migraine with prolonged aura when the main symptoms are a decrease of consciousness, headache and vomiting. The following are two examples.

Case 1

A 6-year old girl had several attacks of confusion, decreased level of consciousness, headache and nausea when she was watching the TV. The diagnosis between migraine and an epileptic fit was unclear. Her standard EEG was normal. When she was filmed in front of the TV set, she had an attack lasting 20 minutes (this was stopped by using valproate IV infusion). The EEG abnormalities appear at the beginnig of the attack and are typical of occipital seizure *(Fig. 11a, b)*. The patient presented idiopathic photogenic occipital epilepsy (Guerrini, 1995).

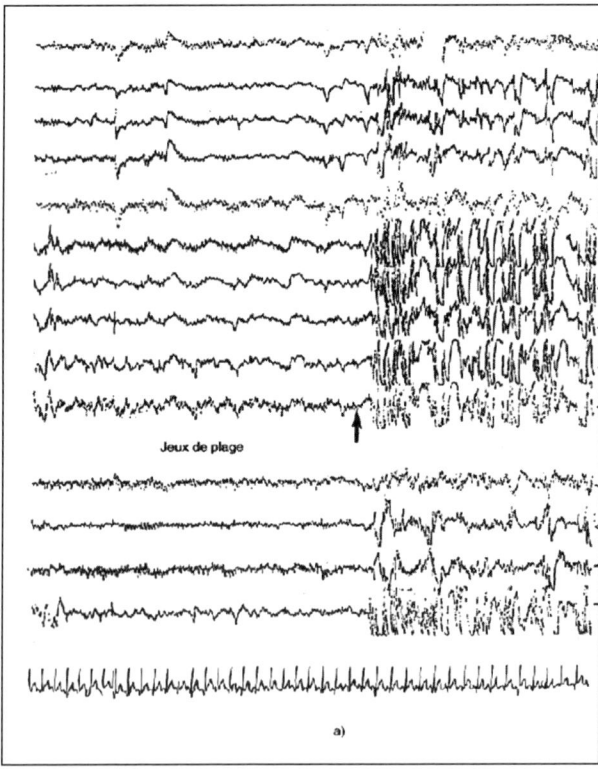

Figure 11a. Photoparoxysmal response to video game on TV screen (arrow).

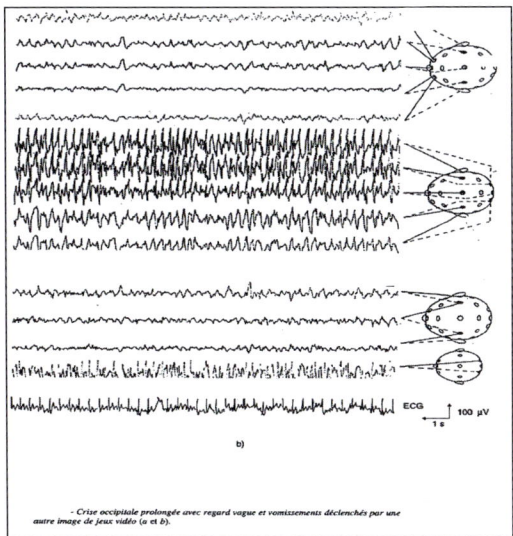

Figure 11b. The photoparoxymal response is followed by occipital status associated with prolonged rythmic occipital ictal activity.

Case 2

A young 2.5-year old boy had attacks of decreased level of consciousness, several times a week, with vomiting at awakening, during approximately 45 minutes. There were no motor automatisms or eye deviation. He had right occipital spikes and waves on standard EEG. The diagnosis result was between BTM associated with seizures (Camfield, 1978) or only occipital epilepsy with recurrent status. During a 72 hours EEG video, we have recorded an attack which was clearly an occipital epileptic status with focal rythmic activity at the beginning of the attack *(Fig. 12a, b, c)* followed by post ictal non rhythmic slow waves. The MRI showed a right occipital perinatal ischemic lesion.

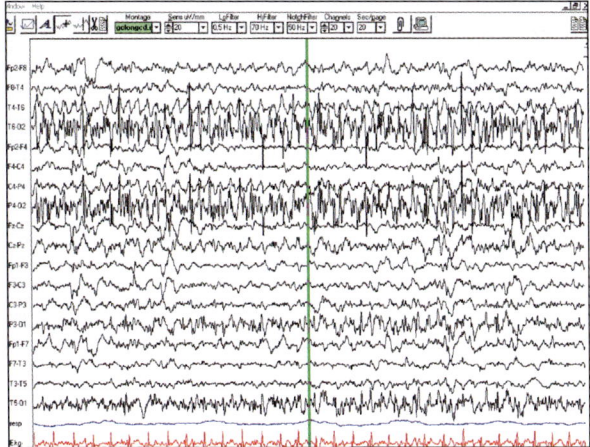

Figure 12a. Ictal rhythmic fast activity in right occipital area.

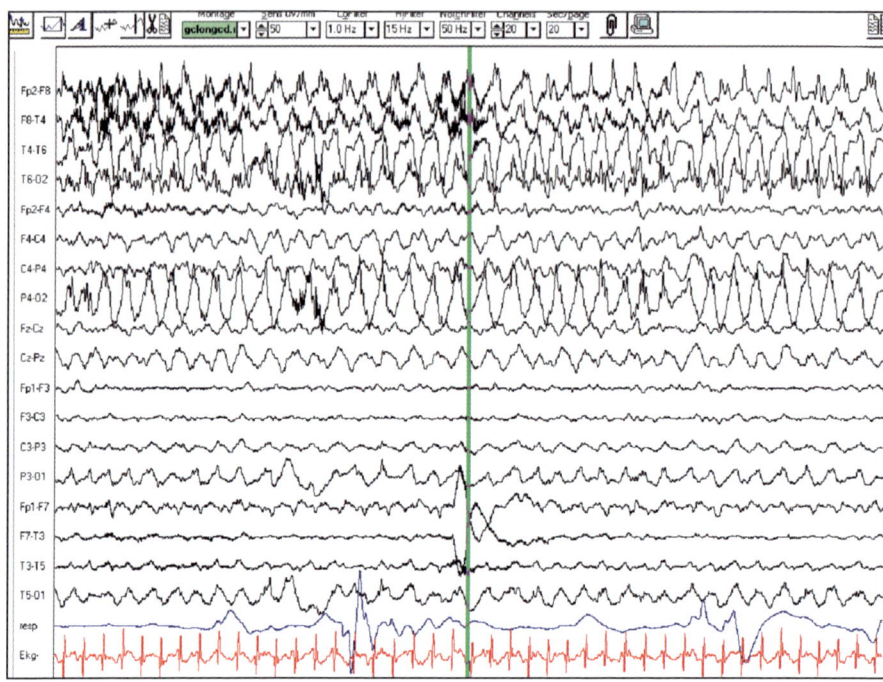

Figure 12b. The ictal rhythmic activity is slower and higher.

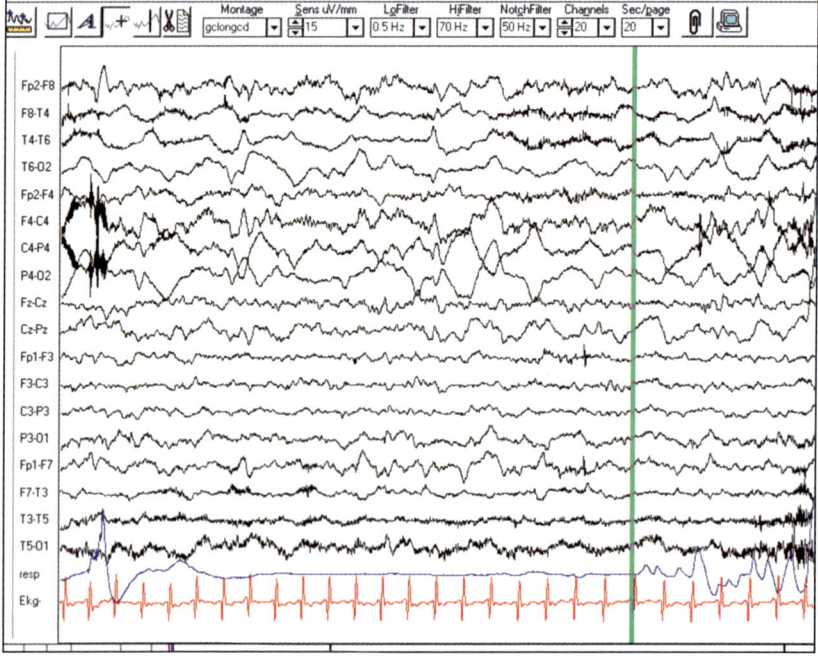

Figure 12c. Post ictal non rhythmic slow waves abnormalities.

Conclusion

The two conditions, prolonged migraine aura and epileptic seizure, may be clearly distinguished by EEG and sometimes TCD. The different sequences of EEG and TCD abnormalities can be used as a diagnostic tool to differentiate migraine aura from some occipital epileptic seizures or even transient ischemic strokes. Epileptic seizures are associated with immediate focal EEG abnormalities and TCD in most cases remains normal. In transient ischemic stroke, the EEG remains normal at D1 and D2. In migraine with prolonged aura, the EEG abnormalities appear after several hours and TCD may be altered when there is a cerebral hemispheric dysfunction.

Acknowledgement: The author thanks Richard Medeiros, Rouen University Hospital medical editor, for editing the manuscript.

References

- Andersen AR, Friberg L, Olsen TS, *et al*. Delayed hyperemia following hypoperfusion in classic migraine: single photon emission computed tomographic demonstration. *Arch Neurol* 1988; 45: 154-9.

- Beaumanoir A. An EEG contribution to the study of migraine and of the association of migraine and epilepsy in childhood. *In*: Andermann F, Beaumanoir A, Mira L, Roger J, Tassinari, eds. *Occipital Seizures and Epilepsies in Children*. London: John Libbey, 1993: 101-10.

- Bowyer SM, Aurora KS, Moran JE, *et al*. Magnetoencephalographic fields from patients with spontaneous and induced migraine aura. *Ann Neurol* 2001; 50: 582-7.

- Camfield PR, Metrakos K, Andermann F. Basilar migraine, seizures and severe epileptiform EEG abnormalities. *Neurology* 1978; 28: 584-8.

- Commission on Classification and Terminology of the International League Against Epilepsy (ILAE). Proposal for revised classification of epilepsies and epileptic syndromes. *Epilepsia* 1989; 30: 389-99.

- De Benedittis G, Ferrari Da Passano C, *et al*. CBF changes during headache-free periods and spontaneous/induced attacks in migraine with and without aura: a TCD and SPECT comparison study. *J Neurosurg Sci* 1999; 43: 141-6.

- De Romanis F, Buzzi MG, Assenza S, *et al*. Basilar migraine with electroencephalographic findings of occipital spike-wave complexes: a long-term study in seven children. *Cephalalgia* 1993; 13: 192-6.

- De Romanis F, Buzzi MG, Assenza S, *et al*. Basilar migraine with electroencephalographic findings of occipital spikewave complexes: a long-term study in seven children. *Cephalalgia* 1993; 13: 192-6.

- Emery ES. Acute confusional state in children with migraine. *Pediatrics* 1977; 60: 110-4.

- Gascon G, Barlow C. Juvenile migraine, presenting as an acute confusional state. *Pediatrics* 1970; 45: 628-35.

- Goadsby PJ. Migraine physiopathology. *Headache* 2005; 45: S14-S24.

- Guerrini R, Dravet C, Genton P, *et al*. Idiopathic photosensitive occipital lobe epilepsy. *Epilepsia* 1995; 36: 883-91.

- Haas DC, Laurie H. Trauma-triggered migraine: an explanation for common neurological attacks after mild head injury. *J Neurosurg* 1988; 68: 181-8.

- Hadjikhani N, Sanchez del Rio M, Wu O, *et al*. Mechanisms of migraine aura revealed by functional MRI in human visual cortex. *Proc Natl Acad Sci USA* 2001; 98: 4687-92.

- Headache Classification Subcommittee of the International Headache Society. The International Classification of Headache Disorders, 2nd ed. *Cephalalgia* 2004; 24 (suppl. 1):1-160.

- Lapkin ML, French JH, Golden GS, Rowan AJ. The electroencephalogram in childhood basilar artery migraine. *Neurology* 1977; 27: 580-3.

- Lauritzen M. Pathophysiology of the migraine aura. The spreading depression theory. *Brain* 1994; 117: 199-210.

- Lauritzen M., Trojaborg W., Olesen J. EEG during attacks of common and classical migraine. *Cephalalgia* 1981; 1: 63-6.

- Olesen J, Friberg L, Skyhoj-Olsen T, *et al*. Timing and topography of cerebral blood flow, aura, and headache during migraine attacks. *Ann Neurol* 1990; 28: 791-8.

- Parain D, Hitzel A, Guégan-Massardier E, *et al*. Migraine with prolonged aura in children: a sequence of EEG slow-wave abnormalities *versus* vascular events. *Cephalalgia* 2007; 27: 1043-9.

- Parain D, Samson-Dollfus D. Electroencephalograms in basilar artery migraine. *Electroencephalogr Clin Neurophysiol* 1984; 58: 392-9.

- Parisi P, Kasteleijn-Nolst Trenite D, Piccioli M, *et al*. Case with atypical childhood occipital epilepsy "Gastaut type": an ictal migraine manifestation with a good response to intravenous diazepam. *Epilepsia* 2007; 48: 2181-6.

- Sánchez del Rio M, Alvarez Linera J. Functional neuroimaging of headaches. *Lancet Neurol* 2004; 3: 645-51.

- Sand T. EEG in migraine: a review of the literature. *Funct Neurol* 1991; 6: 7-22.

- Soriani S, Scarpa P, Arnaldi C, *et al*. Migraine aura without headache and ictal fast EEG activity in an 11-year-old boy. *Eur J Pediatr* 1996; 155: 126-9.

- Woods RP, Iacoboni M, Mazziotta JC. Brief report: bilateral spreading cerebral hypoperfusion during spontaneous migraine headache. *N Engl J Med* 1994; 331: 1689-92.

- Zanette EM, Agnoli A, Cerbo R, *et al*. Transcranial Doppler (TCD) after nitroglycerin in migraine without aura. *Headache* 1991; 31: 596-8.

Epilepsy and familial hemiplegic migraine. Genetic and clinical aspects

Axel Lebas, Évelyne Guégan-Massardier, Lucie Guyant-Maréchal
Rouen

Migraine and epilepsy are two paroxysmal cerebral disorders. In the recent years, the co-occurrence of both disorders in families with Familial Hemiplegic Migraine (FHM) has been described (Haan, 2008), suggesting common physiopathological mechanisms.

FHM is a rare autosomal dominant variant of migraine with aura (MA) (Headache Classification Committee of the International Headache Society, 2004). Typical FHM's aura symptoms include unilateral – rarely bilateral – motor weakness or paralysis, variably associated with typical symptoms of MA (chronologically visual obscuration, sensory symptoms and aphasia) (Thomsen, 2002). Duration of headache is usually prolonged, lasting up to 2 or 3 hours. FHM and MA attacks may co-occur within FHM families. In addition, FHM patients can have severe atypical attacks with signs of diffuse encephalopathy, impairment of consciousness, confusion or coma. Prolonged hemiplegia attacks lasting several days have also been reported.

Mutations in three types of ion channels have been found in FHM families: the α1A subunit of Cav2.1 neuronal voltage-dependant calcium channel, the A1/A2 Na+/K+-ATPase subunit and the neuronal voltage gated sodium SCN1A channel. Genetic-clinical phenotype analyses reveal no specific relationship between the type of channel or mutation and clinical manifestation in FHM families. However, several individuals in FHM1 families had migraine attacks and progressive mild cerebellar signs (Ducros, 1999; Sparado, 2004; Fernandez, 2008). This was not reported in FHM2 or FHM3 families.

This chapter summarizes the current knowledge concerning families in which hemiplegic migraine attacks and epilepsy are associated and explores potential pathophysiologic mechanisms.

Genetic of familial hemiplegic migraine

FHM is genetically heterogeneous. Three genes and one additional locus implicated in FHM have been described, termed FHM 1, 2, 3, 4.

CACNA1A, FHM1 (MIM 141500)

Mutations in the *CACNA1A* gene on chromosome 19p13, encoding the α1A subunit of the Cav2.1 neuronal voltage-dependant calcium channel have been identified in approximated 50% of FHM families (Ophoff, 1996). *CACNA1A* is composed of 47 exons covering 300 kb. Over 18 different missense mutations have been described in FHM1. All of them produce substitutions of amino acids that are situated in important functional regions of the protein, including the pore lining and the voltage sensors. These amino acids are known to be highly conserved residues in α-subunit in different species (Stam, 2008).

CACNA1A channels are multimeric proteins located within the cell membrane. The central pore opens in response to membrane depolarisation, permitting calcium ions influx into the cell. Each channel is formed by a main α1 subunit associated with four auxiliary subunits α2, β, γ, and δ (De Waard, 1996). There are at least 6 classes of α-1 subunits: α-1A, B, C, D, E, and S, which are derived from 6 genes representing members of a gene family. The α1A is abundantly expressed in the brain and in peripheral neurons at the neuromuscular junction. It consists of four repeated domains I-IV, each of which contains 6 transmembrane regions S1-S6 comprising a voltage sensor S4 and a pore loop between S5 and S6. Studies of the functional consequences of *CACNA1A* mutations suggested increase of intracellular Ca^{2+} as a major effect. Mutations modify the density and the gating properties of P/Q-type currents. The functional studies of FHM mutations suggest gain of function of human neuronal Cav2.1 channels. Mutant human $Ca_v2.1$ channels open at lower voltages and more readily than WT channels. Thus, Ca^{2+} influx through mutant channels can occur in response to small depolarisations insufficient to open WT channels.

Two other autosomal dominant disorders are caused by *CACNA1A* mutations: episodic ataxia type 2 (EA2) and spinocerebellar ataxia type 6 (SCA6) (Denier, 1999; Ophoff, 1996). Autosomal dominant SCA6 is due to expansions of CAG repeat at the 3' terminus of the *CACNA1A* gene resulting in truncating protein. Four point mutations in the *CACN1A1* gene have also been described in SCA6 families (Jen, 1998). The *CACNA1A* mutations described in EA2 have not been reported in FHM families (Stam, 2008). The mechanism of ataxia is postulated to be due to abnormal protein synthesis.

ATP1A2, FHM2 (MIM 602681)

Mutations of the *ATP1A2* gene on chromosome 1q23 encoding the A1A2 Na+/K+-ATPase subunit cause FHM2 (De Fusco, 2003). The FHM2 phenotype may be associated with paroxysmal cerebellar ataxia (Thomsen, 2007), psychiatric and cognitive problems (Castro, 2008), prolonged hemiplegia (Jen, 2007), fever, meningism and coma (Deprez, 2008). The Na+/K+-ATPase is an integral plasma membrane enzyme that couples the hydrolysis of ATP to the countertransport of Na+ and K+ across the membrane. It is a key regulator of cellular ion homeostasis and is important to several cellular functions, including control of cell volume and pH, and the generation of action potentials. The Na+/K+-ATPase protein is composed of 3 heteromeric subunits, the α or catalytic subunit, the β or regulatory subunit, and the γ subunit, whose function is unknown. There are 4 α subunit genes of which 1-3 are expressed in the central nervous system.

A small part of the α subunit is exposed on the extracellular side of the membrane. Both the amino and carboxy termini are located intra-cellularly. The FHM2 mutations are located in the intracellular ATP catalytic domain and in the extracellular loops involved in α-subunit binding and ion conduction (Jorgensen, 2003). The p.Met731Thr (M731T) and p.Arg689Gln (R689Q) mutations are present in the large loop between transmembrane domains M4 and M5. This loop harbors the ATP-binding and hydrolase domains of the protein. The p.Met731Thr (M731T) is located in a highly conserved sequence in the junction region, essential for the interactions between the catalytic and membranous cation binding sites during cation translocation. The p.Arg689Gln (R689Q) residue is located in the same important functional hydrolase domain but outside the junction sequence. The p.Leu764Pro (L764P) mutation is located in the same intra-cellular loop.

Loss of Na+/K+ ATPase function may depolarize neurons and rendering them hyperexcitable, which may facilitate seizures. Furthermore, increase of extracellular K+ will facilitate cortical spreading depression (CSD), the likely mechanism for migraine aura. Increase of intracellular Na+ will enhance intracellular Ca2+ through Na+-Ca2+ exchanger function, which will also facilitate the cortical spreading depression.

SNC1A, FHM3 (MIM 609634)

A missense mutation, p.Gln1489Lys (Q1689L), in the neuronal voltage gated sodium channel gene *SNC1A* on chromosome 2q24 was found in 3 FHM families in which *CACNA1A* and *ATP1A2* gene mutations were excluded (Dichgans M, 2005). SCN1A is a voltage-gated ion channel essential for the generation and propagation of action potentials, chiefly in nerve and muscle. Voltage-sensitive sodium channels are heteromeric complexes consisting of a large central pore-forming glycosylated α subunit and 2 smaller auxiliary beta subunits.

Mutations in *SCN1A* cause generalized epilepsy with febrile seizures plus (GEFS+) and severe myoclonic epilepsy of infancy (Ceulemans, 2004; Claes, 2001; Escayg, 2000). The p.Gln1489Lys (Q1489L) mutation is not associated with epilepsy. A second mutation, p.Leu1649Gln (L1649Q), was identified in another family (Vanmolkot, 2007). No seizure was reported. Both FHM3 mutations lead to impaired fast inactivation and predict enhanced neuronal excitation (Dichgans, 2005; Vanmolkot, 2007). However, the reason why these two mutations cause pure FHM is unknown.

FHM4 (MIM 607516)

FHM4 locus on chromosome 1q31, was described in an American family with FHM, without epilepsy, linked to chromosome 1q31 (Gardner, 1997). The causative gene has not been yet identified.

Familial hemiplegic migraine and epilepsy

The first report of an association between FHM attacks and epileptic seizures concerned a child (Kramer, 1997) who experienced between the age of 6 and 12, partial tonic-clonic seizures concomitant to 5 HM attacks. The side of the body affected by the seizure always corresponded to the side of the hemiplegia. No genetic studies were available for this family at the time of the diagnosis.

Epileptic disorders and HM attacks may be considered in 4 different situations:

– Seizures can occur during HM attacks. When reported, epileptic phenomena are partial, generalized or secondarily generalized. Seizures can be the initial manifestation or appear during the course of an HM attack, as seen in FHM2 families (Ducros, 1997) and in FHM1 families (Ducros, 2001). This sequence indicates a close temporal link between epileptic seizures and FHM attacks. Since these first observations, numerous descriptions of epileptic seizures were reported at the beginning or during HM attacks. Data are shown in *tables I and II*, respectively for FHM1 and FHM2 families. To our knowledge, seizures concomittant to HM attacks were not reported with mutations of FHM3.

Table I. *CACN1A1* mutations associated with occasional epileptic seizures during HM attacks

Mutations	N	Age	Clinical symptoms	References
p.Tyr1385Cys Y1385C	1	31 y-o	One partial seizure with left-sided tonic movements and brief recurrent episodes of tonic eye deviation	(Vahedi, 2000)
p.Trp1684Arg W1684R	2	Ns	Partial or generalized seizures during 7 of 8 HM attack (subject 1) One partial (tonic eye deviation) and one generalized tonic seizure (subject 2)	(Ducros, 2001)
p.Arg1668Try R1668W	1	Ns	One partial seizure (same side as hemiplegia)	(Ducros, 2001)
p.Thr666Met T666M	1	15 y-o	One episode of tonic-clonic seizures	(Kors, 2003)
p.Ile1710Thr I1710T	1	14 y-o	Three status epilepticus (2 partial, 1 generalized) during FHM attacks	(Beauvais, 2004)
p.Ser218Lys S218L	1	17 y-o	Paroxysmal activity on EEG during the acute phase of his HM attack	(Chan, 2008)

Ns: not specified ; N: number of reported subjects; y-o: year-old.

– Seizures can occur in the same individual without any temporal link with FHM attacks. The coexistence of both types of paroxysmal events was mainly described in FHM2 (*Table III*), occasionally in FHM1 (*Table IV*) and in FHM3 families (*Table V*).

– Seizures and HM attacks can both occur in the same family but not in the same individual. A large Dutch family has been reported with FHM attacks and a benign familial infantile epileptic syndrome. Some individuals had both disorders, while others had only migraine attacks or epileptic seizures. Genetic studies revealed a new FHM2 mutation point (Vanmolkot, 2003).

Table II. *ATP1A2* mutations associated with occasional epileptic seizures during HM attacks

Mutations	N	Age	Clinical symptoms	References
p.Arg834Gln R834Q	1	8 y-o	One generalized tonic-clonic seizure 2 hours after the onset of his first migraine attack	(Ducros, 1997; Riant, 2005)
p.Met829Arg M829R	1	5 y-o	Partial seizures 2 hours after the onset of his first HM attack. Clonic movements of both arms predominating on the hemiplegic side	(Ducros, 1997; Riant, 2005)
p.Gly301Arg G301R	5	Various	Partial motor seizures in 1 individual, generalized tonic-clonic seizures in 4 individuals concomittant with FHM attacks	(Spadaro, 2004)
p.Gly615Arg G615R	1	4 y-o 7 y-o	Two severe FHM attacks with Sz: 1 with a generalized seizure 1 with a status epilepticus	(Vanmolkot, 2006)
p.Gly900Arg G900R	1	22 y-o	Status epilepticus at day 5 after the onset of a severe HM attack with coma	(Deprez, 2008)
p.Arg548Cys R548C	1	5 y-o 12 y-o	Four brief generalized tonic seizures at the beginning of the most severe HM attack	(Lebas, 2008)

N: number of reported subjects; y-o: year-old; Sz: seizure.

– Genes involved in familial hemiplegic migraine are also involved in epileptic disorders. Some mutations involving the three FHM genes have been shown to cause epilepsy with no concomitant manifestations of FHM. The locations of the mutation sequences were different from those reported in FHM. The p.R1820stop mutation of *CACNA1A* gene was reported in one case of childhood absence epilepsy (Jouvenceau, 2001), a usually benign form of generalized epilepsy during childhood. In that case, the epileptic syndrome was composed of day-time absence seizures associated with generalized tonic-clonic seizures. This patient had also episodic ataxia and developed later a fixed cerebellar syndrome. Numerous mutation sequences among *SCN1A* were previously identified as the underlying genetic factor of about 70% of patients with Dravet syndrome, and in some families with febrile and afebrile seizures (Scheffer, 1997; Wallace, 1998). These mutations were different from those described in FHM3 families (Dichgans, 2005; Vanmolkot, 2007).

Table III. *ATP1A2* mutations associated with a human epilepsy outside HM attacks in FHM2 families

Mutations	N	Age	Clinical symptoms	References
p.Leu764Pro L764P	3	2 y-o 3 y-o 6 y-o	Seizures in 3 subjects Favorable course with remission Seizures types undefined	(De Fusco, 2003; Marconi, 2003)
p.Trp887Arg W837R	2	Ns	Partial secondary generalized seizures starting with visual disturbances. Favorable course under treatment (phenobarbital and phenytoin)	(De Fusco, 2003; Marconi, 2003)
p.Asp718Asn D718N	1	4 y-o 7 y-o	Generalized tonic-clonic seizures	(Jurkat-Rott, 2004)
p.Pro979Leu P979L	1	From 8 m to 2 y	Recurrent generalized tonic-clonic seizures from age 8 m to 2 y	(Jurkat-Rott, 2004)
p.Thr378Asn T378N	4	From 18 m to 3 y	Complex phenotype with FHM and alternating hemiplegia of childhood in 4 members Generalized tonic-clonic seizures with or without fever	(Swoboda, 2004)
p.Gly615Arg G615R	3	Ns	Childhood epilepsy	(Vanmolkot, 2006)
p.Gly900Arg G900R	5	From adolescence	Partial seizures (4 patients). Generalized seizures (1 patient).	(Deprez, 2008)
p.Asp999His D999H	6	Ns	Febrile seizures (2) Childhood absence epilepsy (2) Generalized epileptic seizures (1) Partial, secondary generalized epileptic seizures (1)	(Fernandez, 2008)
p.Arg548Cys R548C	1	From 6 to 10 y	Childhood absence epilepsy	(Lebas, 2008)

Ns: not specified; N: number of reported subjects; y-o: year-old; y: year; m: month; numbers in parentheses: number of reported subjects.

Table IV. *CACN1A1* mutations associated with a human epilepsy outside HM attacks in FHM1 families

Mutations	N	Age	Clinical symptoms	References
p.Arg689Gln R689Q	4	Infantile period	Generalized infantile seizures	(Terwindt, 1997; Vanmolkot, 2003)
p.Ile1710Thr I1710T	2	5 y-o	Several episodes of complex partial seizures. One generalized tonic-clonic seizure. Benign course with AED after 11 y-o	(Kors, 2004)
		1,5 y-o	Complex partial seizure Several generalized tonic-clonic seizures Favorable outcome after AED until 9 y-o	(Kors, 2004)
p.Ser218Lys S218L	2	5 y-o	Five separate generalized tonic-clonic seizures triggered by mild head trauma. Favorable outcome without AED	(Chan, 2008)
		From 2 y to 4 y	Simple febrile seizures during infancy and a secondary generalized tonic-clonic seizure at age 4 y during a febrile illness	(Chan, 2008)

AED: anti-epileptic drugs; N: number of reported subjects; y-o: year-old; y: year.

Table V. *SCN1A* mutations associated with a human epilepsy outside HM attacks in FHM3 families

Mutations	N	Age	Clinical symptoms	Reference
p.Gln1489Lys Q1489L	3	Childhood 3 m Childhood	Attacks of hemiplegic migraine and epileptic seizures during infancy Febrile convulsion (1) Febrile convulsion (1) Benign focal epilepsy	Dichgans, 2005

N: number of reported subjects; m: month; Numbers in parentheses: number of reported subjects.

Conclusion

Migraine and epilepsy are two paroxysmal disorders both related to dysfunction of ion exchanges. Dysfunction of ion exchanges play a key role in the genesis of neuronal network synchronization and cortical spreading depression. The co-occurrence of seizures and FHM attacks argues for a direct causal link between these two episodic disorders. Migraine and epilepsy share common characteristics: both are paroxysmal events with transient abnormalities on EEG and anti-epileptic medications may have benefit in both. Direct evidence of a shared pathophysiology, however, requires further elucidation.

References

- Beauvais K, Cavé-Riant F, De Barace C, et al. New *CACNA1A* gene mutation in a case of familial hemiplegic migraine with status epilepticus. *Eur Neurol* 2004; 52: 58-61.

- Castro M, Nunes B, de Vries B, et al. Two novel functional mutations in the Na+,K+-ATPase alpha2-subunit ATP1A2 gene in patients with familial hemiplegic migraine and associated neurological phenotypes. *Clin Genet* 2008; 73: 37-43.

- Ceulemans BPGM, Claes LRF, Lagae LG. Clinical correlations of mutations in the *SCN1A* gene: from febrile seizures to severe myoclonic epilepsy in infancy. *Pediatr Neurol* 2004; 30: 236-43.

- Chan Y, Burgunder J, Wilder-Smith E, et al. Electroencephalographic changes and seizures in familial hemiplegic migraine patients with the CACNA1A gene S218L mutation. *J Clin Neurosci* 2008; 15: 891-4.

- Claes L, Del-Favero J, Ceulemans B, et al. De novo mutations in the sodium-channel gene SCN1A cause severe myoclonic epilepsy of infancy. *Am J Hum Genet* 2001; 68: 1327-32.

- De Fusco M, Marconi R, Silvestri L, et al. Haploinsufficiency of ATP1A2 encoding the Na+/K+ pump alpha2 subunit associated with familial hemiplegic migraine type 2. *Nat Genet* 2003; 33: 192-6.

- De Waard M, Gurnett CA, Campbell KP. Structural and functional diversity of voltage-activated calcium channels. *Ion Channels* 1996; 4: 41-87.

- Denier C, Ducros A, Vahedi K, et al. High prevalence of *CACNA1A* truncations and broader clinical spectrum in episodic ataxia type 2. *Neurology* 1999; 52: 1816-21.

- Deprez L, Weckhuysen S, Peeters K, et al. Epilepsy as part of the phenotype associated with ATP1A2 mutations. *Epilepsia* 2008; 49: 500-8.

- Dichgans M, Freilinger T, Eckstein G, et al. Mutation in the neuronal voltage-gated sodium channel SCN1A in familial hemiplegic migraine. *Lancet* 2005; 366: 371-7.

- Ducros A, Denier C, Joutel A, et al. The clinical spectrum of familial hemiplegic migraine associated with mutations in a neuronal calcium channel. *N Engl J Med* 2001; 345: 17-24.

- Ducros A, Denier C, Joutel A, et al. Recurrence of the T666M calcium channel *CACNA1A* gene mutation in familial hemiplegic migraine with progressive cerebellar ataxia. *Am J Hum Genet* 1999; 64: 89-98.

- Ducros A, Joutel A, Vahedi K, et al. Mapping of a second locus for familial hemiplegic migraine to 1q21-q23 and evidence of further heterogeneity. *Ann Neurol* 1997; 42: 885-90.

- Escayg A, MacDonald BT, Meisler MH, et al. Mutations of *SCN1A*, encoding a neuronal sodium channel, in two families with GEFS+2. *Nat Genet* 2000; 24: 343-5.

- Fernandez DM, Hand CK, Sweeney BJ, Parfrey NA. A novel *ATP1A2* gene mutation in an Irish familial hemiplegic migraine kindred. *Headache* 2008; 48: 101-8.

- Gardner K, Barmada MM, Ptacek LJ, Hoffman EP. A new locus for hemiplegic migraine maps to chromosome 1q31. *Neurology* 1997; 49: 1231-8.

- Haan J, Terwindt GM, van den Maagdenberg AMJM, Stam AH, Ferrari MD. A review of the genetic relation between migraine and epilepsy. *Cephalalgia* 2008; 28: 105-13.

- Headache Classification Committee of the International Headache Society. The International Classification Of Headache Disorders. *Cephalalgia* 2004; 24 (suppl. 1): 22-136.

- Jen JC, Klein A, Boltshauser E, et al. Prolonged hemiplegic episodes in children due to mutations in ATP1A2. *J Neurol Neurosurg Psychiatry* 2007; 78: 523-6.

- Jen JC, Yue Q, Karrim J, Nelson SF, Baloh RW. Spinocerebellar ataxia type 6 with positional vertigo and acetazolamide responsive episodic ataxia. *J Neurol Neurosurg Psychiatry* 1998; 65: 565-8.

- Jorgensen PL, Hakansson KO, Karlish SJD. Structure and mechanism of Na,K-ATPase: functional sites and their interactions. *Annu Rev Physiol* 2003; 65: 817-49.

- Jouvenceau A, Eunson LH, Spauschus A, *et al*. Human epilepsy associated with dysfunction of the brain P/Q-type calcium channel. *Lancet* 2001; 358: 801-7.

- Jurkat-Rott K, Freilinger T, Dreier JP, *et al*. Variability of familial hemiplegic migraine with novel A1A2 Na+/K+-ATPase variants. *Neurology* 2004; 62: 1857-61.

- Kors EE, Haan J, Giffin NJ, *et al*. Expanding the phenotypic spectrum of the *CACNA1A* gene T666M mutation: a description of 5 families with familial hemiplegic migraine. *Arch Neurol* 2003; 60: 684-8.

- Kors EE, Melberg A, Vanmolkot KRJ, *et al*. Childhood epilepsy, familial hemiplegic migraine, cerebellar ataxia, and a new CACNA1A mutation. *Neurology* 2004; 63: 1136-7.

- Kramer U, Lerman-Sagi T, Margalith D, Harel S. A family with hemiplegic migraine and focal seizures. *Eur J Paediatr Neurol* 1997; 1: 35-8.

- Lebas A, Guyant-Maréchal L, Hannequin D, Riant F, Tournier-Lasserve E, Parain D. Severe attacks of familial hemiplegic migraine, childhood epilepsy and ATP1A2 mutation. *Cephalalgia* 2008; 28: 774-7.

- Marconi R, De Fusco M, Aridon P, *et al*. Familial hemiplegic migraine type 2 is linked to 0.9Mb region on chromosome 1q23. *Ann Neurol* 2003; 53: 376-81.

- Ophoff RA, Terwindt GM, Vergouwe MN, *et al*. Familial hemiplegic migraine and episodic ataxia type-2 are caused by mutations in the Ca2+ channel gene *CACNL1A4*. *Cell* 1996; 87: 543-52.

- Riant F, De Fusco M, Aridon P, *et al*. ATP1A2 mutations in 11 families with familial hemiplegic migraine. *Hum Mutat* 2005; 26(3): 281.

- Scheffer IE, Berkovic SF. Generalized epilepsy with febrile seizures plus. A genetic disorder with heterogeneous clinical phenotypes. *Brain* 1997; 120 (Pt 3): 479-90.

- Spadaro M, Ursu S, Lehmann Horn F, *et al*. A G301R Na+/K+ -ATPase mutation causes familial hemiplegic migraine type 2 with cerebellar signs. *Neurogenetics* 2004; 5: 177-85.

- Stam AH, van den Maagdenberg AM, Haan J, Terwindt GM, Ferrari MD. Genetics of migraine: an update with special attention to genetic comorbidity. *Curr Opin Neurol* 2008; 21: 288-93.

- Swoboda KJ, Kanavakis E, Xaidara A,, *et al*. Alternating hemiplegia of childhood or familial hemiplegic migraine? A novel ATP1A2 mutation. *Ann Neurol* 2004; 55: 884-7.

- Terwindt GM, Ophoff RA, Lindhout D, *et al*. Partial cosegregation of familial hemiplegic migraine and a benign familial infantile epileptic syndrome. *Epilepsia* 1997; 38: 915-21.

- Thomsen LL, Eriksen MK, Roemer SF, Andersen I, Olesen J, Russell MB. A population-based study of familial hemiplegic migraine suggests revised diagnostic criteria. *Brain* 2002; 125: 1379-91.

- Thomsen LL, Kirchmann M, Bjornsson A, *et al*. The genetic spectrum of a population-based sample of familial hemiplegic migraine. *Brain* 2007; 130: 346-56.

- Vahedi K, Denier C, Ducros A, *et al*. *CACNA1A* gene de novo mutation causing hemiplegic migraine, coma, and cerebellar atrophy. *Neurology* 2000; 55: 1040-2.

- Vanmolkot KRJ, Babini E, de Vries B, *et al*. The novel p.L1649Q mutation in the *SCN1A* epilepsy gene is associated with familial hemiplegic migraine: genetic and functional studies. Mutation in brief. Online. *Hum Mutat* 2007; 28: 522.

• Vanmolkot KRJ, Kors EE, Hottenga J, *et al*. Novel mutations in the Na+, K+-ATPase pump gene *ATP1A2* associated with familial hemiplegic migraine and benign familial infantile convulsions. *Ann Neurol* 2003; 54: 360-6.

• Vanmolkot KRJ, Stroink H, Koenderink JB, *et al*. Severe episodic neurological deficits and permanent mental retardation in a child with a novel FHM2 ATP1A2 mutation. *Ann Neurol* 2006; 59: 310-4.

• Wallace RH, Wang DW, Singh R, *et al*. Febrile seizures and generalized epilepsy associated with a mutation in the Na+-channel beta1 subunit gene *SCN1B*. *Nat Genet* 1998; 19: 366-70.

Treatments: overlap between migraine and epilepsy in children

Jean-Christophe Cuvellier, Louis Vallée
Lille, France

Migraine and epilepsy are considered quite different clinical entities and typically diagnosis is based on well-defined and widely accepted international classification standards. Migraine is the most frequent recurrent headache syndrome in children. The prevalence of migraine headache in children in the general population ranges between 2.7% and 17%. About 3% to 5% of school-aged children experience attacks of migraine, and this proportion gradually increases through adolescence. It is estimated to affect nearly 20% of adolescents, making it the most common cause of headache in pediatric patients. Initially, there is a slight male preponderance; however, through adolescence there is a shift toward female predominance, which remains through adulthood. Ten and half million children worldwide are estimated to have active epilepsy. Over the past 15 years, syndrome-oriented clinical and EEG diagnosis, and better aetiological diagnosis, especially supported by neuroimaging, has helped to clarify the diversity of epilepsy in children, and has improved management. Ion channel defects can underlie both benign age-related disorders and severe epileptic encephalopathies with a progressive disturbance in cerebral function. Several new antiepileptic drugs have been recently introduced but have provided controversial therapeutic benefits.

It is well-known that children with infantile idiopathic epilepsy (epilepsy with rolandic or occipital paroxysms, absence epilepsy) show concomitant migraine in up to 60% of the cases, and 4% to 8% of the people with migraine suffer from epileptic seizures. In pediatric migraine patients, generalized or focal sharp waves, slow waves, spike and wave discharges, periodic lateralized epileptiform epileptiform discharges, benign focal sharp waves, and centrotemporal spikes have been reported with or without an accompanying seizure. Nevertheless studies concerning the comorbidity migraine and epilepsy have mainly been performed in adult populations, and there are few data available in children and adolescents. Yamane *et al.* (Yamane, 2004) studied the comorbidity between headache and epilepsy in 50 children with epilepsy and found that 43.5% and 20% of them had headaches and migraine, respectively. They noted a frequent association between headaches and seizures (39%). The study by Stevenson *et al.* (2006) revealed a higher prevalence of migraine in pediatric epilepsy patients (14.7%) than in the general population. These data suggest that epilepsy and migraine are comorbid conditions. Preliminary genetic studies have already provided clues about the pathogenesis of some clinical forms of epilepsy and migraine, suggesting a channel function alteration underlying both types of diseases. More recently it was suggested that neuronal hyperexcitability might explain the comorbidity of migraine (especially migraine with aura) and epilepsy, and an increased occurrence of spreading depression might be the link between these 2 comorbid conditions.

Treatment of pediatric migraine includes an individually tailored regimen of both nonpharmacological and pharmacological measures (Wasiewski, 2001). The nonpharmacological modalities include life-style adjustments (*e.g.*, sleep hygiene, caffeine moderation, dietary adjustments, and a regular exercise program), reassurance, stress management, biofeedback, and other biobehavioral therapies. The mainstay of treatment is intermittent oral analgesics, but up to 30% of young migraineurs experience such frequent and disabling attacks that they require daily prophylaxis with a variety of medications, including antiepileptic drugs (AEDs). Although many agents have been used as preventive medications for migraine headache both in children and adults, there is a paucity of controlled clinical research in the treatment of childhood and adolescent migraine. Thus there is little evidence to support the efficacy of prophylactic drugs. This statement is equally true for antiepileptic drugs for migraine prophylaxis. Consequently, physicians use anecdotal experiences or extrapolated adult information when selecting medicines for treatment. Prophylactic pharmacological treatment could be considered when headache frequency exceeds 4 episodes per month and/or the attacks are so severe or prolonged that they interfere with school or normal activities. Drugs commonly used for migraine are calcium antagonists, β-blockers and pizotifen. The reviews available so far have concluded that behavioural therapies seemed more effective than prophylactic drug regimens.

The United States Food and Drug Administration has approved so far 2 antiepileptic drugs for adult migraine prophylaxis. In August of 2004, topiramate became the second antiepileptic drug, along with valproate, to be approved for the treatment of migraine prophylaxis in adults. To date, no antiepileptic drugs are approved for this purpose in children younger than 12 years. The approvals are based upon large, randomized clinical trials in adults, and consequently, do not extend to children and adolescents. Although antiepileptic drugs are frequently employed for a variety of nonepileptic disorders in children and adolescents, including migraine, well-designed studies in these populations are lacking. Information on antiepileptic drug use in pediatric migraine comes mainly from small, open-label trials and case reports. According to the four-tiered classification scheme for therapeutic evidence devised by the American Academy of Neurology, most pediatric publications on this topic merit the lowest rating (class IV), and thus, do not allow for the formulation of policy regarding the use of antiepileptic drugs in pediatric migraine. Moreover, it should be noted that the lack of controlled trials results in a literature bias towards favorable results. Despite these limitations, it is important for the practicing clinician to be aware of the evidence underlying the use of antiepileptic drugs in pediatric migraine.

Given the current views regarding the pathophysiology of migraine as involving a primary neuronal initiation of a cascade of events and subsequent propagation through "spreading depression" across the cerebral cortex, anticonvulsants pose an extremely intriguing, although incompletely defined, role. Sodium valproate, divalproex sodium, gabapentin, levetiracetam and zonisamide have been studied in children, but topiramate is the only AED to have been studied in a controlled fashion in children and adolescents.

We chose to divide the following review in three parts. The first one will deal with the available studies concerning pediatric migraine prophylaxis with "conventional" antiepileptic drugs in both migraine without aura and migraine with aura. The second one will review the available information about the use of drugs not considered as routine antiepileptic drugs but known to possess demonstrable anticonvulsant effects, such as flunarizine, nimodipine and magnesium. In the last part, we will envisage the use of antiepileptic drugs in the prophylaxis of 2 childhood periodic syndromes, formerly known as migraine equivalents: abdominal migraine and cyclic vomiting syndrome.

"Conventional" antiepileptic drugs

Clinical trials evaluating "conventional" AEDs are shown in *Table I*.

Sodium valproate and divalproex sodium

Valproic acid (VPA) was approved for migraine prophylaxis by the Food and Drug Administration in 1996. It is usually used in the form of divalproex sodium, an oligomeric complex composed of sodium valproate and VPA in a 1:1 ratio. The mechanism of action of VPA in migraine prophylaxis may be related to facilitation of γ-aminobutyric acid (GABA)-ergic neurotransmission, decreasing the activation of serotonergic cells, and attenuation of neurogenic inflammation. Divalproex sodium may exert its protective effect by suppressing migraine-related cortical events, perivascular parasympathetic activity, or trigeminal nucleus caudalis activity. Alternatively, it may attenuate nociceptive neurotransmission or suppress neurogenic inflammation. Thus, divalprocx sodium may alter migraine genesis at several sites along the pathway from stimulus to headache pain.

Double-blind, placebo-controlled studies and a variety of open trials have documented that VPA is an effective preventive treatment for adult migraine. No double-blind, placebo-controlled study is available in children and adolescents, where we only dispose of open label studies and one comparative study.

Ashrafi *et al.* (2005) conducted a multicenter randomized clinical trial to compare the effect of sodium valproate in pediatric migraine prophylaxis with that of propranolol, but there was no control group and no blinding in patients and care provider physicians to therapeutic agents. One hundred and twenty patients with migraine without and with aura, according to International Headache Society (IHS) criteria, aged from 7 to 16 years were randomly divided in 2 groups of A and B, whether they were being treated with sodium valproate or propranolol, respectively. Three phases of baseline period (phase I; 4 weeks), titration and adjustment period (phases II; 4 weeks) and fixed-dose treatment period (phase III; 2 months) had been designed. A total of 57 patients (mean: 10 ± 2.3 years) in group A and 58 patients (mean: 9.7 ± 2.7 years) in group B completed all phases of the trial. Seventy-two percent ($P < 0.05$) of group A patients and 69% ($P < 0.05$) of group B patients showed a greater than 50% headache frequency reduction.

Table I. Overview of antiepileptic drugs migraine prophylaxis studies in children and adolescents

Drug Author (year)	Design	Dose	N*	Age (y)	Results
VPA					
Caruso (2000)	OL	15-45 mg/kg/d	42	7-16	Improvement in 78.5%
Pakalnis (2001)	R	3.1-32.9 mg/kg/d	23	7-17	Improvement in 62.5%
Serdaroglu (2002)	OL	500-1,000 mg/d	10	9-17	Improvement in 90%
Freitag (2002)	DB R PC parallel	500-1,000 mg/d	202	16-69	Extended-release effective
Ashrafi (2005)	R parallel	10-40 mg/kg/d	57	7-16	Improvement in 72%
GBP					
Belman (2001)	R	5.5-30 mg/d	18	6-17	Improvement in 83%
TPM					
Hershey (2002)	OL	2.07 mg/kg/d	97	13.6 (a)	Improvement in 81%
Winner (2005)	DB R PC parallel	15-200 mg/d	162	6-15	Improvement in 32%
Campistol (2005)	OL	1.8-6 mg/kg/d	24	6-14	Improvement in 88%
Winner (2006)	DB R PC parallel	100 or 200 mg/d	49	12-16	Improvement in 63% (100 mg), 65% (200 mg)
Lakshmi (2007)	DB R PC	100 mg/d	42	8-14	Improvement in 95.2%
Lewis (2007)	DB R parallel	25 or 100 mg/d	14	6-18	Improvement in 86%
Brandes (2004)	DB R PC	50, 100 or 200 mg/d	468	12-65	Improvement in 47%
Silberstein (2006)	DB R PC	50, 100 or 200 mg/d	469	12-65	Improvement in 52%
Shaygannejad (2006)	DB R crossover vs. VPA 200-400 mg/d	25-50 mg/d	64	14-57	Improvement in both groups; no difference between drugs
LVT					
Miller (2004)	R	250-1,500 mg/d	19	11.9 (a)	Improvement in 89%
Vaisleib (2005)	OL	NR	19	6-19	Improvement in 89%
DeSouza (2005)	R	500-1,500 mg/d	15	11-19.5	Improvement in 80%
Pakalnis (2007)	OL, prospective	20-40 mg/kg/d	20	10-17	Improvement in 90%
ZNS					
Pakalnis (2006)	R	5.8 mg/kg/d (m)	12	9-17	Improvement in 67%

VPA: valproic acid; TPM: topiramate; GBP: gabapentin; LVT: levetiracetam; ZNS: zonisamide; (a): average; DB: double-blind; NR: not reported; OL: open-label; PC: placebo-controlled; R: randomized; RCR: retrospective chart review.
* Number of patients completing the study

Moreover both drugs showed efficacy in reducing headache duration (52% of group A and 53% of group B patients, respectively) and severity (56% of group A and 64% of group B patients had less severe headache at least for one grade after prophylactic therapy with sodium valproate and propranolol, respectively). Further more 61% of group A and 67% of group B of cases had a better response to rescue medications and 21% of group A and 17% of group B of them became headache free. There was no significant difference in all previously mentioned therapeutic effects between 2 groups ($P < 0.05$).

In the open label trial by Caruso et al. (2000), 42 patients with a mean age of 11.3 ± 2.8 years (range: 7 to 16 years), who had IHS migraine with or without aura, were treated with divalproex sodium and were followed during 6.6 to 20.9 months (mean: 13.7 months). All previous prophylactic medications had been discontinued. Their baseline frequency ranged between 1 to 4 migraines per month during the 6 months preceding the study. Chronic daily headache (CDH) was excluded. The primary efficacy analysis was based on percentage of headache relief after divalproex sodium prophylactic treatment over a 4-week period, with the goal of achieving a 50% or greater reduction in headache frequency. Dosage of divalproex sodium was increased until less than one headache per month was achieved. Final divalproex sodium dosage ranged from 15 mg/kg/day to 45 mg/kg/day. Of the 42 patients, 34 (80.9%) successfully discontinued their abortive medications. After 4 months of treatment, 50% and 75% headache frequency reduction was seen in 33 (78.5%) and 6 (14.2%) patients, respectively (all $P < 0.05$). Four (9.5%) of them even became headache-free. Moreover, 34 (80.9%) discontinued their abortive medications, and 39 (92.8%) reported significantly less need for abortive headache medications after 6 months of treatment with divalproex sodium. Eighty-one percent of patients had improved school attendance and less restriction of daily activities. Twenty-nine experienced adverse events, the most frequent adverse event (14/29) being gastrointestinal upset. Other adverse events included weight gain, somnolence, tremor, and dizziness. Four patients had mild increases in results of liver function tests.

Another open label study was conducted by Serdaroglu et al. (Serdaroglu, 2002), in 10 children (6 boys, 4 girls) aged 9-17 years (13.6 ± 3.2 years) with migraine according to IHS criteria. They were treated with sodium valproate at daily doses which ranged between 500 and 1,000 mg (mean dose: 750 mg), the final dose being adapted according to blood levels. Severity was measured using a visual analog scale (VAS; 0 to 5) and a numerical rating scale (NRS; 0 to 5). Both headache severity and frequency were reduced. Mean severity was reduced from 6.8 ± 1.8 to 0.7 ± 1.2 (VAS; $P = 0.000$) and from 4.7 ± 0.5 to 0.6 ± 1.1 (NRS; $P = 0.000$) between baseline (8 weeks) and the end of the 12 weeks of the study treatment. Mean headache attacks frequency was reduced from 6.0 ± 4.2/month to 0.8 ± 1.9/month ($P = 0.002$) and mean duration of headache attack was reduced from 5.5 ± 3.9 hours to 1.1 ± 2.5 hours following treatment ($P = 0.001$). The drug's therapeutic effect was first evident at about the fourth week. In 2 cases, headache attacks recurred after the cessation of valproate, and therapy was restarted. Headache control lasted for 6 months following cessation of the drug in 8 subjects. Side effects included dizziness, drowsiness, and increased appetite, but no serious side effects were noted in this small study. After study completion, 2 patients restarted medication because headaches recurrence. The other patients experienced benefit for 6 additional months after cessation of therapy.

Pakalnis *et al.* (2001) reviewed the charts of 23 patients (13 girls) fulfilling IHS criteria for migraine, 7-17 years (mean: 12.4 years), suffering from 3 to 24 attacks per month, both to assess the effectiveness and safety of divalproex sodium when used in migraine prophylaxis, and to evaluate associated comorbid epilepsy (n = 6) or behavioural/psychiatric disorders (n = 7). Standardized headache questionnaires and diaries were used. Concurrent psychotropic medications were noted. All patients were of normal intelligence. Divalproex sodium doses ranged from 250 to 1.125 mg/day (3.1-32.9 mg/kg/day). Fifteen patients (65.2%) had a greater than 50% reduction in headache frequency, with 6 (26%) of them becoming headache-free. Only greater than 50% improvement was evaluated. When considering the different groups, one may notice that patients with concurrent psychiatric disorders did not improve with divalproex, whereas patients with comorbid epilepsy or migraine alone had a statistically significant favorable response ($P = 0.002$). No significant difference in dose was found between the groups. Four patients had side effects requiring discontinuation (weight gain, lethargy, anorexia, alopecia – one each). This study suggests that divalproex may have a selective efficacy in the prevention of migraine and is well tolerated with low doses and serum levels. It raises the question whether a differential positive response to divalproex in migraine therapy could be influenced by a concurrent comorbidity, and the possibility of a differential biochemical reactivity in each case.

Fusco *et al.* (Fusco, 2002) followed 3 patients, aged 9, 12 and 15 years, fulfilling the IHS criteria for migraine with and without aura. They were treated with low doses of sodium valproate (10 mg/kg/day) during 6 months. All patients experienced a greater than 50% reduction in their attacks frequency, during the following year. The duration of attacks decreased from more than 2 hours to less than 2 hours and intensity from severe to moderate to mild. The treatment enabled a reduction in the use of symptomatic medications. The plasma VPA concentration was always below 50 mg/dl. VPA was generally well tolerated: in only one subject was the drug stopped because of weight gain. The authors suggested that VPA might thus be effective at a low dosage.

Mendizabal *et al.* (2002) reported on 2 adolescents treated by extended-release divalproex sodium during 6 months. In addition to a good efficacy and tolerance, the authors showed an improvement in the quality of life of both patients, as demonstrated by the Migraine Specific Quality of Life Questionnaire.

See also the study by Shaygannejad *et al.* (2006) comparing topiramate and VPA which is discussed in the next section (Topiramate).

Topiramate

Topiramate (TPM) is a neuromodulatory compound with stabilizing properties that was initially introduced for the management of epilepsy. It has been demonstrated to modify several receptor-gated and voltage-sensitive ion channels, including voltage-activated Na^+ and Ca^{2+} channels and non-N-methyl-D-aspartate (NMDA) receptors, these last ones implicated in the pathophysiology of both epilepsy and migraine. The mechanisms of action of TPM may stem from its broad pharmacological profile. For example, its ability to enhance GABA-mediated neurotransmission, inhibit voltage-activated Ca^{2+} channels and block glutamate-mediated excitatory neurotransmission likely explain why it is efficacious in the prophylactic management of migraine. The effectiveness of TPM as a prophylactic agent was confirmed in several double-blind, placebo-controlled pediatric studies.

Winner et al. (Winner, 2005), summarized the results of an outpatient study conducted at 17 medical centers throughout the United States. Included subjects had to be aged 6 to 15 years, met the IHS criteria for migraine with or without aura, weigh more than 20 kg, and experience 3-10 migraine days per month for the 3 months prior to the screening and during the 4-week prospective baseline phase. They were randomized in a 2:1 ratio to receive TPM or placebo. The study consisted in a baseline phase (4 weeks), followed by a titration phase during which TPM was slowly increased to a target dose of 2 to 3 mg/kg/day, or maximum-tolerated dose, whichever was less, with the maximum dose allowed being 200 mg/day. Then followed the maintenance phase which lasted 12 weeks. The primary efficacy variable was the change in mean number of migraine days per month (28 days) during the double-blind phase relative to the 4-week prospective baseline phase for each treatment group. One-hundred and fifty-seven subjects were included in the intention to treat (ITT) population, defined as randomized subjects who had received at least one dose of study medication and had at least one postbaseline efficacy assessment, and a total of 131 children completed the study (per-protocol population); of these, 108 were treated with TPM. Primary outcome measure was the reduction of migraine days per month in each treatment group of the ITT population. The subgroup of the ITT population which received TPM at a mean average daily dose of 2.0 mg/kg/day during the maintenance period, had a mean age of 11.3 ± 2.5 years, a mean weight of 50.6 ± 24.9 kg; the male/female ratio was 50.9/49.1. During the double-blind phase, in the ITT population, relative to the 4-week prospective baseline, there was a reduction of 2.6 ± 2.6 migraine days per month for TPM-treated subjects compared with a mean reduction of 2.0 ± 3.1 days per month for placebo-treated subjects, for over the entire double-blind phase. This result only approached statistical significance ($P = 0.061$). The same reduction in mean monthly migraine days was statistically significant in the per-protocol population (2.8 ± 2.4 days vs. 2.2 ± 2.1 days, $P = 0.033$). The percentage of TPM-treated ITT subjects showing $> = 50\%$ reduction in monthly migraine days during the double-blind phase was 54.6% compared with 46.9% in the placebo group and was not statistically significant. However, the percentage of TPM-treated subjects showing $= 75\%$ reductions in monthly migraine days (32.4%) was significantly greater than that of the placebo group (14.3%, $P = 0.020$). In addition, during the last 28 days of treatment, the mean number of monthly migraine was reduced by 3.1 ± 2.6, as opposed to 2.4 ± 2.8 in the placebo group ($P = 0.023$). TPM was well tolerated, with the most common adverse events occurring at greater incidence than in the placebo group being: upper respiratory tract infection (19.4%), anorexia (13.0%), weight decrease (10.2%), gastroenteritis (9.3%), paresthesias (8.3%), and somnolence (8.3%). The majority of adverse events were mild to moderate in severity. Discontinuation rates due to adverse events were low: 6.5% for the TPM group and 4.0% for the placebo group. Serious adverse events occurred in 4 TPM-treated subjects and included infection (n = 2), severe migraine (n = 1), and suicidal ideation (n = 1). The mean change from baseline in body weight was - 0.7 ± 3.9 kg for subjects treated with TPM and 1.4 ± 2.6 kg for those receiving placebo. In conclusion, although the relatively greater reduction by TPM-treated subjects in the ITT population experienced a relatively greater reduction in migraine days per month, this result did not achieve statistical significance. Other end points, including the proportion of patients experiencing at least a 75% reduction in migraine days, and reduction in migraine days and responder rates during the last 28 days of treatment, were significantly in favour of TPM-treated subjects. That the reduction was more evident in the last 28 days of treatment may indicate that it may take a few weeks before treatment with TPM reach its maximum efficacy.

The same author (Winner, 2006) recently pooled the data from the patients aged 12 to 17 years who participated in 3 large, similarly designed placebo-controlled, double-blind trials, each which individually enrolled a limited sample of pediatric patients, and was able to perform a post hoc subset analysis of the efficacy and safety data from these patients. A total of 51 patients, aged 12 to 17 years, with an established history of migraine with or without aura, as defined by the IHS diagnostic criteria for migraine, were enrolled in the original 3 trials, at a total of 150 sites. Patients were to have had between 3 and 12 migraine attacks, and no more than 14 headache days per 28 days during the 3 months prior to the screening and during the 4-week prospective baseline phase. TPM was administered at the dosages of 50, 100 or 200 mg a day for 26 weeks. The analysis was based on a small population and used post hoc methods, which limits the conclusions that can be drawn. However, the analysis of the data drawn from the 49 patients, aged 14 ± 2 years, which were included in the ITT population, revealed that daily treatment with TPM 100 (n = 13) and 200 mg (n = 13) for 26 weeks reduced statistically significantly monthly migraine frequency from baseline of 63% ($P = 0.02$) and 65% ($P = 0.04$), respectively, compared with placebo (16%). Results from treatment with 50 mg/day did not reach statistical significance ($P = 0.07$). TPM treatment reduced the mean number of monthly migraine days by 4 and 5 days for TPM 100, and 200 mg/day doses, respectively, and placebo treatment reduced this by 1 day. Similarly, TPM treatment reduced the percentage from baseline of days of acute (rescue) medication use by 59%, 54%, and 67%, for the 50, 100, and 200 mg/day doses, respectively, compared with 42% for placebo. TPM 200 mg/day did not appear to offer greater efficacy than 100 mg/day. Treatment was generally well-tolerated, although adverse events were most frequent in the 200 mg/day dose group, which did not appear to confer additional efficacy as opposed to the dosage of 100 mg a day.

The recent study by Lakshmi *et al.* (2007) was a randomized, double-blind, placebo-controlled trial involving 44 children who were randomized (in a 1:1 ratio) to receive either placebo or TPM (titrated to 100 mg a day) for 12 weeks. Patients had a diagnosis of migraine without aura, according to the IHS diagnostic criteria, and experienced 2 or more headaches per month during the 3 preceding months. Primary outcome measures were the reduction in migraine frequency and severity; secondary outcome measures included number of analgesics taken and the functional disability. Migraine monthly frequency decreased from 16.14 ± 9.35 at baseline to 4.27 ± 1.95 at the end of the study in the TPM group as compared with a decrease from 13.38 ± 7.78 to 7.48 ± 5.94 in the placebo group ($P = 0.025$). The percentage of TPM-treated subjects showing > 50% reduction in monthly migraine days during the double-blind phase was 95.2% as opposed to 52.4% in the placebo group ($P = 0.002$). The Pediatric Migraine Disability Assessment (PedMIDAS) also decreased significantly ($P = 0.003$) as did school absenteeism ($P = 0.002$). Side effects were rated mild to moderate, did not cause any dropouts and included weight-loss, with a mean loss of 0.3 kg (81%), paresthesias (23.8%), loss of appetite (23.8%), decreased concentration (19%), sedation (19%) and abdominal pain (14.3%).

Several case studies and open-label studies also suggest the effectiveness of TPM for use as a potential prophylactic treatment for migraine in children. The study by Campistol et al. (2005) was an open, prospective, multicenter observational study of case series, which included 24 patients (13 boys), aged 10.4 ± 2.2 years. TPM was prescribed at the mean dosage of 3.5 ± 1.7 mg/kg/d for 4 months. Most patients had taken previous prophylactic treatments without success: flunarizine (54%), cyproheptadine (41%), propranolol (20%). There was a reduction in the mean frequency of migraines from initiation of TPM (3.6 ± 2.7 migraines/month) on subsequent visits at 2 months (2.9 ± 2.2 migraines/month) and 4 months (2.7 ± 2.4 migraines/month; $P = 0.061$), but which was not significant. The migraine severity at 2 months and 4 months was significantly reduced when compared with the initial visit ($P < 0.0001$ and $P = 0.001$, respectively). Similarly, the number of patients reporting severe attacks dropped from 11 (45.8%) at baseline to 1 (5.3%) after 4 months of TPM treatment. Although the dosage of TPM was higher (mean dosage: 3.5 ± 1.7 mg/kg/day with a maximum of 200 mg/day) than that reported in the previous series, it was well tolerated by the majority of patients.

The study by Hershey et al. (2002) suffered from the fact that different types of headache were mixed. It included ninety-seven children with frequent headache; of these, 79.4% met the IHS criteria for migraine, 8.2% with aura. "Using clinical impression for the diagnosis", 96.9% had migraine and 8.2% had migraine with aura. They were prescribed TPM for headache prevention (2.0 ± 0.7 mg/kg/day). Forty-seven percent of the patients had CDH. The mean headache frequency was reduced from 16.5 ± 10.0 to 8.7 ± 10.8 days per month at the last follow-up (320 ± 65 days; $P < 0.001$). Severity and duration of headache also were reduced. Headache disability improved, with a reduction of PedMIDAS score from 36.0 ± 42.3 to 10.9 ± 16.9 at the last follow-up ($P < 0.001$). Most patients tolerated TPM well. The most common side effects reported were cognitive changes (12.5%), weight loss (5.6%), and sensory symptoms (2.8%). A possible bias of this study is that 50.7% of patients were on additional prophylactic medication (most often amitriptyline or divalproex).

Two abstracted retrospective reports (Younkin, 2002) of the use of TPM for children headache included 31 patients in whom there was a mean decrease in headache frequency of 70% at a mean dose of 76 mg per day with 7 patients reporting sedation, cognitive slowing, loss of appetite, and weight loss effects. A study by Ferreira et al. (2002) described 35 patients with migraine in whom there was a mean decrease in headache frequency of 77% at a mean dose of 138 mg/day. Thirty-three percent of patients experienced mild adverse events including decreased appetite, paresthesia and weight loss.

The study by Shaygannejad et al. (2006) comparing TPM and VPA was not conducted exclusively within the pediatric population but included patients as young as 14 years. This study demonstrated that treatment with TPM (50 mg daily) and VPA (400 mg daily) both significantly reduced migraine headache, with a significant decrease in duration, monthly frequency, and intensity of headache in both groups.

Basilar-type migraine is a form of migraine with aura characterized by the onset of transient bulbar (e.g., vertigo, dizziness, diplopia, dysarthria) and/or bilateral sensorimotor (e.g., leg paresthesias, cortical visual disturbances) symptoms, followed by a migraine headache. Lewis and

Paradiso (2007) conducted a double-blind, parallel-group, dose comparison study which included subjects with basilar migraine according to the second edition of the International Classification of Headache Disorders (ICHD-II) and > 4 migraines/month. They were randomized to receive either 25 mg per day or 100 mg per day of TPM in a 1:1 ratio. The primary endpoint was reduction in average monthly migraine days over the entire double-blind phase relative to the prospective baseline period. Among several secondary efficacy outcomes, migraine disability was also assessed using PedMIDAS. Fourteen patients completed the double-blind phase, with 7 patients each randomized to the 25-mg group (6 girls, 1 boy, mean age, 13.57 ± 1.72 years, average number of both migraine with aura, including basilar-type migraine, and migraine without aura attacks per month, 8) and the 100-mg group (4 girls, 3 boys, mean age, 13.29 ± 2.93 years, average number of all migraine attacks per month, 5). No other preventive therapies were permitted. The average monthly migraine days were 4.5 (25 mg) and 4.8 (100 mg) and the average duration and severity were similar between the 2 groups. There was a reduction of 3.97 migraine days per month from the prospective baseline to treatment maintenance phase ($P < 0.001$) without significant difference ($P = 0.86$) between the 2 groups: the reduction in mean monthly migraine rate during the double-blind treatment phase relative to baseline was 2.9 (64.4%) for the 25-mg and 3.6 (75.0%) for the 100-mg TPM-treated group. For the target headache subtype, basilar-type migraine, the reduction in mean monthly rate during the double-blind treatment phase relative to baseline was 2.5 (74.24%) and 2.3 (82.8%) for the 25-mg and 100-mg TPM-treated groups, respectively. Disability was significantly reduced with the baseline disability scores falling by a mean of 29.2 points on the PedMIDAS. Numbness and tingling in the face and hands were the most common adverse events, but no patient withdrew from the study and no serious adverse events were reported. Thus, regardless of treatment dose (25 mg *vs.* 100 mg), patients had significantly fewer monthly migraine days and experienced significant improvement in migraine-associated disability and quality of life as measured by the PedMIDAS, but there was no placebo arm and the sample size was small.

Gabapentin

Gabapentin (GBP) is an anticonvulsant agent structurally related to the inhibitory neurotransmitter GABA. Although GBP was developed as a structural analog of GABA that would penetrate the blood-brain barrier (unlike GABA) and mimic the action of GABA at inhibitory neuronal synapses, GBP does not interact with GABA receptors, is not converted to GABA, and is not an inhibitor of GABA uptake or degradation. Thus, its precise mechanism of action has not been elucidated and GBP must exert its effects on migraine genesis through an alternative mechanism other than GABA neurotransmission.

There is only one study, which is a retrospective one, moreover reported in abstract form, conducted by Belman *et al.* (2001), involving 18 children aged 6 to 17 years (mean: 12.25 years), treated with GBP. Migraine prophylaxis was indicated because of prolonged or frequent headaches (more than 3 severe attacks per month) that interfered with school, sports, or social activities. Dosage was slowly increased during the first 2 to 3 weeks of therapy to 5.5 to 30 mg/kg/day (mean: 15.1 mg/kg/day) with twice-daily dosing for all but 3 children. Headache frequency and severity was decreased by more than 50% in 15 children. Three children stopped medication because of dizziness, sleep disturbance, or no effect. The authors concluded that GBP appeared to be well-tolerated and effective in migraine prevention in children.

Levetiracetam

Levetiracetam (LVT), a pyrrolidine derivative, is an anticonvulsant agent that is structurally unrelated to other currently available anticonvulsants. The mechanism of anticonvulsant action of LVT is unknown and does not appear to be related to any known mechanisms involved in excitatory or inhibitory neurotransmission. But, given its excellent tolerability profile, and using the rational that virtually all commercially available anticonvulsants have shown efficacy in the treatment of migraine, this drug has recently been evaluated for this use, both in adult and pediatric migraine prevention.

In the first trial (Miller, 2004), charts of 19 pediatric patients (9 girls and 10 boys; mean age, 11.9 years, range, 3-17 years; mean body weight, 54.9 kg, range, 12-100 kg) who had been treated by LVT for migraine were retrospectively reviewed. IHS migraine and IHS migraine with aura accounted for 63.2% and 15.8% of the sample respectively, with the remainder corresponding to abdominal migraine (2 patients), migraine and CDH (1 patient), and "atypical migraine, possible cluster headache" (1 patient). Most patients (89.5%) had severe migraine. Eleven of these children previously had used other prophylaxis medications. Four patients were on concomitant prophylaxis with TPM, GBP, atenolol, or amitriptyline (1 each). Mean duration of LVT treatment was 4.1 months (range, 1.25 to 7 months). Doses ranged from 125 to 750 mg twice daily. Mean monthly headache attacks frequency was reduced from 6.3 (standard deviation (SD), 3.8; confidence interval, 4.4 to 8.1) to 1.7 (SD, 2.7; confidence interval, 0.4 to 3.0) ($P < 0.0001$). Ten patients (52.6%) became headache free and 7 patients (36.8%) had less severe and less frequent headaches. LVT eliminated nausea and vomiting in 7 patients (36.8%) and abdominal migraine in 1 patient (10.5%). Sixteen patients (82.4%) reported no side effects while on LVT. Two patients discontinued LVT due to side effects: asthenia/somnolence and dizziness in one, irritability, hyperactivity and hostile behaviour in the other.

The second study (Pakalnis, 2007) was a prospective but an open-label one and sample was small. Patients were started on a LVT dosage of 20 mg/kg/day divided twice a day and dosage could be increased to 40 mg/kg/day if necessary. Efficient dosage was carried on 2 months. Twenty patients (5 girls and 15 boys; mean age, 10.65 years, range, 10-17 years), 6 of whom had IHS migraine with aura, completed the study. Mean duration of migraine was 3.15 years (range, 1 to 11 years). Mean monthly headache frequency was reduced from 6.0 ± 1.8 to 2.0 ± 1.9 ($P < 0.001$), with 4 patients (20%) becoming headache free. PedMIDAS decreased from 45.6 ± 31.7 at baseline to 12.1 ± 6.8 with LVT treatment ($P < 0.001$). Eighteen patients (90%) showed a greater than 50% monthly headache frequency reduction from baseline. LVT was generally well tolerated and no patients discontinued drug due to side effects. Three patients had side effects: behavioural changes, including irritability and aggressivity in 2 patients, mild memory problems according to parent's subjective report in 1 patient.

Two abstracted reports of the use of LVT for children headache are available. The first study (DeSouza, 2005) involved 15 adolescent patients (aged 11-19.5 years) with chronic headaches (73% migraines). During a 6-week period, mean headache frequency decreased from 6.8 attacks per month (range 4-30) prior to therapy to 1.5 attacks per month under LVT (range 1-4). The final average dose was 660 mg/day (500 to 1,500 mg/day). Two patients became headache free and 10 reported significant improvement. This response was seen approximately 4-6 weeks after therapy initiation. One patient had no improvement and one experienced more headaches. Fatigue, dizziness, and mood changes were reported by 4 patients. The second study (Vaisleib, 2005) evaluated LVT in 30 patients (aged 6-19 years) over 10 weeks. Patients experienced at least 2 attacks per week prior to therapy. Of 19 subjects who completed the study, 3 became headache free, 8 had a greater than 75% reduction, and 6 had a greater than 50% reduction in frequency and severity. Fifteen subjects had a greater than 75% reduction in their PedMIDAS score. Four patients withdrew because of lack of efficacy and 2 patients experienced worse headaches. One patient withdrew due to seizures and another one withdrew due to delusions and violent behaviour. Mean headache frequencies were not provided, but evaluation of the PedMIDAS was a study strength.

Zonisamide

Zonisamide (ZNS) is a sulphonamide compound thought to block sodium channels and facilitate serotoninergic pathways. Pakalnis *et al.* (2006) reviewed the charts of 12 pediatric patients (8 girls, 4 boys; mean age, 13.5 years, range, 10-17 years) fulfilling IHS criteria for episodic (n = 6) or chronic migraine (n = 6) over a 1-year interval (the remaining 4 patients had CDH of primarily chronic tension type). They had received ZNS therapy for headache prophylaxis, with duration of follow-up ranging from 3 to 18 months. All patients had previously failed at least 2 prior therapeutic medication trials for their headaches, and they had from 2 to 30 headache days per month. While significance was not reported, 8 patients (66.7%) had a greater than 50% headache frequency reduction from baseline. Seven of these patients had episodic migraine. Average ZNS dose used by these positive responders was 5.8 mg/kg/day. All negative responders had CDH. ZNS was generally well tolerated. Only 2 patients discontinued medication, because of weight loss and behavioural changes (one each).

Non-conventional antiepileptic drugs

Flunarizine

Flunarizine is a calcium channel blocker which can modulate neurotransmission and has anticonvulsant properties which were first demonstrated by Desmedt *et al.* (1975) using maximal electroshock or pentetrazole models in rats and maximal electroshock in mice. It is well documented that flunarizine enhances the anticonvulsive activity of a majority of conventional and potential antiepileptics, *e.g.*, VPA, carbamazepine, phenytoin, among others, against maximal electroshock-induced seizures in mice. First clinical evidence for the antiepileptic activity of flunarizine was reported by Declerck and Wauquier (Overweg, 1990). In a clinical trial of 47 adult patients with intractable epilepsy, flunarizine being added to the existing antiepileptic medication, 33 patients had less seizures on flunarizine, 9 had more, and 5 were unchanged. Trials that included children showed similar results to those conducted in adult patients. Flunarizine has also been shown to reduce attack frequency in migraine headaches. It has been used for paediatric migraine prophylaxis and more than one randomized, placebo-controlled, double-blind study has demonstrated its effectiveness. The main mechanism of flunarizine in prevention of recurrent migraine is most likely to be the neurogenic effect in influencing the release of neurotransmitter such as dopamine and met-enkephalin and by blocking calcium and sodium channels

Two studies involving the use of flunarizine in pediatric migraine prophylaxis had been conducted by Sorge *et al.* The first one (Sorge, 1985) was a randomised, double-blind, placebo-controlled, parallel-group study. Diagnosis of migraine rested on Vahlquist criteria (1955). The 48 participants (age range, 7 to 14 years) randomised were divided in 2 groups, group A (n = 24, 14 girls, aged 10.58 ± 3.25 years, 3 classic migraine, 21 common migraine, migraine duration 3.17 ± 1.78 years) and group B (n = 24, 13 girls, aged 10.70 ± 3.29 years, 3 classic migraine, 21 common migraine, migraine duration 2.32 ± 1.52 years). Patients of group A were instructed to take flunarizine 5 mg/day at night for 12 weeks and patients of group B were on placebo. Forty-two patients completed the study. The mean percentage reduction of headache frequency was 65.94% ($P < 0.001$) and the reduction of mean headache duration was 51.05% ($P < 0.05$) *versus* corresponding values in the placebo group of respectively 32.47% ($P < 0.01$) and 16.62% (not significant (NS) at 0.05 level). At the end of the trial the mean frequency of attacks was significantly lower in the flunarizine group than in the control group ($P < 0.001$). The main disadvantage of flunarizine might be the delay of therapeutic efficacy, which peaked at the third month of treatment. The most common side effects were drowsiness, gastrointestinal complaints, weight gain, and fatigue. There were 3 withdrawals in the flunarizine group due to adverse events, and 3 from placebo group due to inadequate pain relief.

The same group published a randomised, double-blind, placebo-controlled, crossover study in 1988 (Sorge, 1988). The design of this study was similar to the previous one (diagnosis of migraine according to Vahlquist criteria, 70 patients randomised, 34/70 males, age range, 5 to 11 years, 7 withdrawals). Following a baseline of 4 weeks, patients of group A (n = 35, 16 girls, aged 10.8 years, migraine duration 2.31 ± 1.5 years) were instructed to take flunarizine 5 mg/day at night for 12 weeks whereas patients of group B (n = 35, 20 girls, aged 10.4 years, migraine duration 2.1 ± 3.1 years) were assigned to take placebo. There followed a washout of 4 weeks, then the crossover period (12 weeks). Group A took placebo and group B flunarizine. Data were represented only graphically. Investigators reported significant reduction in frequency with flunarizine. The frequency of attacks decreased significantly ($P < 0.001$) in group A (flunarizine first) as compared with baseline values from the third month (that is, second month of flunarizine) and remained constant throughout the study also after crossover with placebo. In group B (placebo first) the frequency of headache attacks was significantly reduced ($P < 0.001$) compared with baseline values from the sixth month of the trial (first month of flunarizine) and was maintained throughout the observation period. Similarly duration of attacks was significantly reduced. There were 7 dropouts and 1 patient stopped flunarizine due to excessive daytime sedation. Reported adverse effects were drowsiness and weight gain.

Twenty-one children (10 boys, 11 girls) with an average age of 11.3 ± 2.48 years (range, 7 to 15 years), with a diagnosis of migraine according to the IHS classification, were enrolled in the study by Visudtibhan *et al.* (2004). Nineteen children were initially administered with flunarizine at 5-mg daily. Flunarizine at 10 mg daily was prescribed to the other 2 children who had previous treatment with flunarizine at 5 mg daily in the past 6 months without improvement. Among those who were initially given 5 mg daily, flunarizine was increased to 10-mg daily one month later because of the lack of improvement in 5 patients. Improvement was observed in 14 patients (66%) including 13 of 14 patients who received 5 mg daily and 1 of 7 patients who received 10 mg daily. Five patients (23%) had no recurrent attack. Nine patients (42%) had more than 50% reduction of frequency of migraine and 3 of these had either shorter duration or less intensity of the attack. Clinical improvement was observed between 2 and 4 weeks after initiation of treatment. There was no adverse effect observed.

Flunarizine has also been involved in comparative studies allowing direct active drug-drug comparisons.

Pothmann *et al.* (1987a, b) compared flunarizine with acetylsalicylic acid (ASA) in a randomised parallel-group trial (n = 30) involving 8 weeks of treatment with each intervention. Flunarizine was administered at a dose of 5 mg (for body weight < 40 kg) or 10 mg (for body weight > 40 kg). ASA was administered at a dose of 100 mg (for body weight < 40 kg) or 200 mg (for body weight > 40 kg). ASA decreased monthly frequency of attacks from 7.3 before treatment to 2.1 after treatment. Flunarizine decreased frequency of attacks from 8.0 before treatment to 1.2 after treatment. Eleven on fifteen patients in the ASA group and 10/14 patients in the flunarizine group experienced a 50% or greater reduction in frequency of attacks, but this result was not statistically significant. Adverse events occurred in 5 ASA patients (abdominal pain and nausea in 4) and 8 flunarizine patients (increase in weight and increase in appetite in 5).

Castellana *et al.* (1989) compared flunarizine (5 mg at night) with nimodipine (10 mg 3 times a day) in a randomised open crossover trial (n = 35) involving 30 days of treatment with each intervention. There was a 30-day washout period between periods. Nineteen patients (64% of 30 completers) in both groups had reduction of attacks greater than 50%. Results were presented graphically. The investigators observed moderate side effects only: drowsiness in 4 cases with flunarizine, flushing in 2 cases cases with nimodipine.

Lutschg *et al.* (1990) conducted a randomised parallel-group trial (n = 33) involving 4 months of treatment, either with flunarizine (5 mg at night for body weight 15-25 kg, 10 mg at night for body weight > 25 kg) or propranolol (10 mg 3 times a day for body weight 15-25 kg, 20 mg 3 times a day for body weight > 25 kg). Placebo was given with the flunarizine group to help in blinding (flunarizine was given twice daily while propranolol was given thrice daily). Thirteen of seventeen (76.5%) patients on flunarizine and 12/15 (80%) on propranolol showed a greater than 75% improvement in frequency, which was not statistically significant. Three patients in flunarizine group showed side effects (2 increased tiredness, 1 breathlessness and difficulties of concentration). Five patients in propranolol group showed side effects (4 increased tiredness, 1 pressure behind eyes). Two patients in propranolol group discontinued treatment in 3 months, because of side effects and these settled immediately afterwards.

The study by Lastra Martinez et al. (1990) was a randomised open parallel-group group trial (n = 50) involving 6 months of treatment comparing flunarizine (10 mg once daily) with dihydroergotamine (DHE; 0.5 mg 3 times per day, followed by 1.0 mg 3 times per day, then 1.5 mg 3 times per day). DHE reduced the frequency of attacks (number of attacks per month) from 6.4 (SD, 4.37) before treatment to 2.29 (SD, 2.83) on treatment. Flunarizine reduced the frequency of attacks from 4.16 (SD, 4.01) before treatment to 1.69 (SD, 1.94) on treatment, which was not statistically significant. Reduction of both headaches intensity and duration was NS either. Adverse events were reported by 3 patients with DHE (2 abdominal pain, 1 paraesthesia) and by 5 patients with flunarizine (2 sleepiness, 1 paraesthesia, 2 increased appetite and drinking).

Nimodipine is another Ca^{2+} channel antagonist of the dihydropyridine type which, in addition to its well-documented cerebral vasodilatory effect, also appears to exert anticonvulsant effects, which have been confirmed in experimental models. Several case reports and clinical trials indicate that nimodipine is effective in pediatric patients with seizures refractory to conventional treatment, both by oral and intravenous (IV) route. In addition to the comparative study with flunarizine by Castellana et al. reported above, nimodipine (10-20 mg tid) was also studied in a single controlled, crossover trial (Battistella, 1990) including 37 children ages 7-18 years, but the results were inconsistent between the 2 treatment phases. During the first treatment period, there was no difference between active and placebo. Headache frequency fell from 3.3 to 2.8 attacks per month in the active group and from 3.0 to 2.5 in the placebo group (NS). During the second treatment phase, there was a significant reduction in headache frequency in the nimodipine group, but there was no effect on headache duration. Side effects were limited to mild abdominal discomfort in a little more than 1% of children.

Magnesium

Severe magnesium (Mg) depletion can cause seizures or increase susceptibility to seizure-inducing stimuli. Intravenously infused magnesium exerted an anticonvulsant effect against experimentally-induced epileptic foci in cats and dogs. Oral administration of magnesium has been associated in some cases with an improvement in EEG findings and a reduction in seizure frequency. Low systemic magnesium levels have been demonstrated in the serum, blood cells, saliva, cerebrospinal fluid, and brain of migraineurs compared to nonmigraineur controls, which has led investigators to wonder whether migraine could be a Mg-deficiency disease, at least in part. Magnesium blocked cortical spreading depression of Leão triggered by stimulation of NMDA receptors *in vitro*. Mg may also exert an antimigraine effect by inhibiting platelet hyperaggregability and by relaxing vascular tone. Randomized trials of various Mg salts available in Europe for oral migraine prophylaxis in adults have produced conflicting results.

Wang et al. (2003) conducted a 16-week randomized, double-blind, placebo-controlled, parallel-group trial to assess the efficacy of oral Mg oxide in pediatric migraine. They enrolled children and adolescents of ages 3 to 17 years who reported a 4-week history of at least weekly moderate-to-severe headaches clinically evoking migraine (no IHS criteria) during the previous 4 weeks, to receive either Mg oxide (9 mg/kg per day by mouth divided 3 times a day with food) or placebo for 16 weeks. Eighty-six completed the study (42 received Mg oxide and 44 placebo). One hundred of those enrolled (85%) were between 9 and 16 years of age, inclusive. There was no significant difference between serum total or serum ionized Mg levels comparing the 2 study arms. By ITT analysis, the authors found a statistically significant decrease over time in headache frequency in the Mg oxide group ($P = 0.0037$) but not in the placebo group ($P = 0.086$), although the slopes of these 2 lines were not statistically significantly different from each other ($P = 0.88$). The group treated with Mg oxide had significantly lower headache severity ($P = 0.0029$) relative to the placebo group. Nineteen percent of patients randomized to Mg oxide reported having diarrhea or soft stools, *versus* 7% in the placebo group, which was statistically significant ($P = 0.04$).

Childhood periodic syndromes

Among the clinical entities, formerly known as migraine equivalents, 3 are included by the ICHD-II in childhood periodic syndromes: abdominal migraine (AM), cyclic vomiting syndrome (CVS) and benign paroxysmal vertigo. It must be emphasized that children with childhood periodic syndromes are completely healthy between attacks and, in contrast, are extremely unwell during attacks. The diagnosis of these syndromes is one of exclusion, and involves extensive diagnostic testing to rule out varied etiologies. There is a well-known tendency for childhood periodic syndromes to transform into migraine headaches as the child matures. In AM and CVS, many electroencephalographic abnormalities including generalized discharges have been reported. In some of these reports, patients had loss of consciousness, and some of them were reported as abdominal epilepsy. Of note, especially in benign epilepsy of childhood with occipital paroxysms, vomiting is associated with visual symptoms, partial seizure, and headache. The underlying mechanism of childhood periodic syndromes is not yet understood, but many hypotheses such as mitochondrial cytopathies or ion channelopathies have been discussed.

Cyclic vomiting syndrome

CVS is a disorder characterized by recurrent, severe, discrete, stereotypical attacks of vomiting and intervals of normal health between vomiting episodes averaging 2-4 weeks. The duration of episodes may be from hours to days with spontaneous resolution. The relationship between migraine and CVS is supported by several observations: there is a high prevalence of migraine headache and abdominal pain in paediatric CVS patients, with a higher prevalence of migraine among first-degree relatives of children affected by CVS; migraine headache and CVS share a similar temporal profile of disorder onset and resolution of symptoms; both syndromes share many associated gastrointestinal, sensory and vasomotor symptoms. Published studies have shown the prevalence of migraine headache to be between 30 and 80% in children affected by CVS or AM. The shared therapeutic response of CVS and migraine implies that closely related neurally mediated pathways are responsible for some or all of the symptomatology of these two disorders. Therapy for CVS and AM mainly focuses on preventing attacks with prophylactic medication.

Barbiturates have been recommended for the prophylaxis of cyclic vomiting since the 1950s. The study by Gokhale *et al.* (1997) concerned 14 children (9 girls, 64%), mean age at diagnosis

9.4 years (range, 3.3-13.3 years), mean age at onset, 7.2 years (range, 2.5-12 years), with diagnosed CVS. They were enrolled in the study because they fitted the following criteria: two or more episodes of intractable, self-limiting nausea and vomiting with no identifiable organic cause separated by symptom-free intervals. The vomiting was severe enough to cause dehydration requiring intravenous rehydration in 79% of the children. Abdominal pain was reported in 70% of the patients. There were some arguments in favour of migraine: auras in 43%, headaches in 57% (with 27% fulfilling the diagnostic criteria set for migraine headaches by Prensky), and a family history of migraine headaches in 79%. The patients were placed on daily phenobarbital (PB) administered as a single bedtime dose, with a median dose of 60 mg (range, 30-120 mg, or approximately 2 mg/kg/day). The mean duration of follow-up was 3.8 years (range, 7 months-10.5 years) and the mean duration of PB therapy 2.3 years (range, 0.6-6.3 years). Eleven patients (79%) had ultimately complete resolution of their symptoms, and 3 had marked improvements with infrequent attacks of reduced severity. Thus all 14 patients demonstrated clinical response to PB therapy. The only side effects associated with long-term PB administration were behavioural: hyperactivity or disruptive behavior at school. Dose reduction in 2 patients ameliorated the behavioral disturbances. Only 1 patient required discontinuation of the drug because of side effects. The authors argue that prophylactic, daily, low-dose PB therapy may be a safe and effective therapeutic option in the management of children with cyclic vomiting.

Olmez et al. (2006) reported on the case of a 9.5-year-old female with CVS since 6 years of age. Electroencephalography after sleep deprivation revealed slow and sharp waves during hyperventilation over the posterior sides of the right hemisphere, but no epileptiform activity was recorded. On electroencephalography-video monitoring performed 3 hours immediately after an episode, background activity was normal, but during wakefulness synchronous high-amplitude 3-4 Hz sharp-wave activity for 1-3 seconds was recorded 3 times bilaterally. Neither vomiting nor alteration of consciousness, nor movement of body parts or other signs of a possible seizure were recorded simultaneously. She was started on TPM which was increased to 5 mg/kg/day gradually. She improved. On cessation of TPM, initiated by her parents, she relapsed and improved once more after resumption of treatment.

Palmer and Cameron (2005) reported the case of a teenage boy with CVS who was referred to the anesthesia-run postoperative pain service for symptom management. His symptoms were uncontrolled by oral pizotifen prophylaxis and acute therapy with IV hydration and ondansetron. A continuous low dose IV midazolam infusion, because midazolam IV infusion had been previously reported as effective for postoperative nausea and vomiting, was added to his treatment regimen and resulted in benefit but not total symptom resolution. If one cannot rule out natural resolution as an alternative possibility, it may be possible that clonidine's sympatholytic effects were definitively beneficial or the combination sedative and anxiolytic effects of clonidine and midazolam were responsible.

Abdominal migraine

AM is characterized by recurrent, acute-onset, incapacitating, noncolicky midline abdominal pain – usually periumbilical – and vomiting may be an accompanying feature which may be less severe than in CVS. The key difference between AM and CVS is the common co-existence of abdominal pain and migraine headaches in the patient in AM. The prevalence peaks at 10 years of age and thereafter declines rapidly, even though AM occasionally persists in patients well into adult life.

Kothare et al. (2005) conducted a retrospective analysis of 18 patients seen in a pediatric neurology clinic in Bombay, India, between 2000 and 2002 who satisfied the diagnosis of CVS and AM and who were started on flunarizine. All patients had an extensive diagnostic evaluation to rule out alternate etiologies including MRI brain scan, EEG, abdominal ultrasounds, upper and lower gastrointestinal series, metabolic work up, stool examinations, all of which were normal. Eight children (5 girls and 3 boys) ages 2-8 years (mean age: 3.5 years) had CVS and 10 children (6 girls and 4 boys) ages 4-11 years (mean age: 6 years) had AM. Flunarizine dose was 2.5-10 mg (mean dose: 5 mg/day) in CVS patients and 2.5-15 mg (mean dose 7.5 mg/day) in AM patients. Flunarizine was administered as once a day in 75% and twice a day in 25% patients. Follow up ranged from 6 to 24 months (mean: 13 months). There was a significant reduction in frequency and duration of attacks in both conditions. On flunarizine, there was a 57% reduction in frequency and 44% reduction in duration of attacks of CVS, while there was a 61% reduction in frequency and 51% reduction in duration of attacks of AM. There was a 60% reduction in frequency of headaches on flunarizine in the sixty-four percent of patients with CVS and AM who had also history of episodic recurrent headaches. Twenty-one percent discontinued the medication because of weight gain (15%), or perceived lack of efficacy (6%).

The recent study by Boccia et al. (2005) is equally interesting although the children studied did not correspond to the CVS diagnostic criteria but instead, fitted to the adult Rome II criteria for functional gastrointestinal disorders (FGID). The second part of this study consisted to evaluate 10 migrainous children with associated FGID diagnoses (mean age, 9.8 ± 1.9 years, 7 males), who had indications of preventive treatment according to the American Academy of Neurology Guidelines. These children with migraine received flunarizine 5 mg, as a single daily dose, orally for a period of 2 months. They were compared to a control group of 10 migrainous children without FGID (mean age, 9.2 ± 1.8 years, 6 males) and 9 healthy children (mean age, 8.6 ± 1.7 years, 5 males), who were not in treatment with antimigraine prophylaxis. All patients treated with flunarizine showed a decrease in frequency and duration of migraine attacks. During the study period, subjects treated with flunarizine did not suffer any relevant side-effects. Migrainous children with FGID had significantly more prolonged total gastric emptying time than subjects without FGID. On flunarizine patients had a significant decrease in total gastric emptying time at both 1 ($P < 0.01$) and 2 months ($P < 0.002$) of therapy. The mean frequency of abdominal pain per month was significantly ($P < 0.001$) reduced at 1 month compared with baseline and the mean frequency of vomiting per month was significantly decreased at 1 month ($P < 0.05$) and even more so at 2 months ($P < 0.01$). Finally, the mean frequency of headache per month was significantly reduced only at 2 months ($P < 0.05$), whereas the mean duration of headache was significantly decreased at 1 month. Thus, flunarizine has been shown to decrease the frequency and duration of migrainous episodes as well as the gastrointestinal symptoms.

Clinical implications

At the end of this review, it appears that considerable variation exists in the methodological quality of the different trials examined and that results should be viewed with some caution. It is appropriate, therefore, to stress a number of caveats. A few early studies concerning the use of AEDs for pediatric migraine were done prior to the IHS Classification and used loose criteria to define migraine. Many studies were poorly performed, in the form of open-label, uncontrolled studies in small, nonrandomized samples, or did not provide adequate details of statistical methods. Moreover, a few studies were reported only as abstracts, making proper analysis of the evidence difficult. Further, it is important to stress that the number of trials of each drug is small. Therefore, although the majority of these improperly designed studies have reported positive results, further prospective, randomized, controlled trials are necessary to determine the safety and efficacy of AEDs in the treatment of pediatric migraine. Future trial should also be encouraged to follow the recommendations of the IHS (Tfelt-Hansen, 2000) with regard to both trial design and reporting of data.

In this perspective, it must be stressed that the review provides poorly definite evidence for the efficacy of anticonvulsant drugs in the management of childhood migraine. This rejoins one of the concluding statement of the recently published Practice Parameter (Lewis, 2004), asserting that "the safety and efficacy of currently available medications used to treat migraine headaches in adults need to be established in children and adolescents" and that "It is essential that multicentered, placebo-controlled clinical trials be conducted to assess the safety, tolerability, and efficacy of medications used for the acute and preventive treatment of pediatric and adolescent migraine", remark with which we cannot but fully agree.

This review concluded also, as did also a recent Cochrane Database review of the medical literature (Victor, 2003), that the calcium channel blocker flunarizine is the only agent that has been studied in rigorous controlled trials and found to be effective. Authors also concluded that data from uncontrolled studies suggested 3 antiepileptic drugs (TPM, VPA and GBP) to be effective. Since this review was published, 2 randomized, placebo-controlled trials evaluating TPM in the preventive treatment of pediatric migraine have been carried out (Winner, 2005; Lakshmi, 2007).

Taken together, data from the papers we reviewed suggest that TPM is effective in the preventive treatment of pediatric migraine. Furthermore, TPM dosages, which seem to be effective in the treatment of migraine in children and adolescents (2-3 mg/kg/day) are much lower than those indicated for the treatment of epilepsy (5-9 mg/kg/day). As regards its safety and tolerability, serious adverse effects were very rare, though the risk of depression must be kept in mind. The other most common adverse effects are weight loss, anorexia, cognitive changes and paresthesia. VPA may be efficacious for decreasing migraine frequency and duration in the pediatric population. However, additional trials are needed for confirmation. More information is needed for GBP, LVT, and ZNS considering that most available data are retrospective.

Bearing in mind the limitations invoked by the methodological issues mentioned above, this review nevertheless helps to provide a rational framework for the application of anticonvulsants for the preventive management of migraine headache in real-life clinical practice. A good deal of the published data reviewed above on the use of the AEDs in the treatment of pediatric migraine suggests that each agent may be helpful in some patients. Therefore, the decision to prescribe an AED for any of these conditions must depend on assessment of the potential risks and benefits in the individual patient. It should also be said that one must consider co-morbid conditions, which could help one to choose a drug that will be suitable for both migraine and co-morbid disease or that will not be harmful for the co-morbid condition. For instance, in children with epilepsy and migraine, the use of a single drug to treat both disorders is appealing. It is also evident that the final decision must take into account patient's compliance and preferences. With regard to adverse effects, sometimes we may take advantage of certain drug side effect, *e.g.* the use of TPM in an overweight patient. We will now briefly envisage practical use of these drugs.

Antiepileptic drugs safety profiles

Table II summarizes the adverse effects (AEs) that have been associated with use of the AEDs discussed in this review. Most of them have 2 common AEs: dizziness and somnolence. These AEs were clearly dose related, and most patients developed some degree of tolerance to them over time. Most other AEs in the clinical trials and case series were also dose related, did not lead to discontinuation of treatment, and improved once steady-state levels were achieved and dosing remained constant. It is of note that low initial doses followed by slow titration reduced the incidence and severity of AEs for most of these drugs, with the probable exception of GBP which can be initiated at a higher dose and titrated more quickly than the other AEDs.

Dosing and titration

The starting dose, titration schedule, and target dosage range for each of the drugs are summarized in *Table III*. Therapeutic and/or toxic levels of the newer AEDs have not yet been rigorously defined as they have been for standard AEDs, and serum monitoring of plasma levels is not currently performed on a routine basis. Tailoring of the dose should be dictated on clinical grounds only, taking into account interindividual and intraindividual differences.

Conclusion

In conclusion, topiramate and flunarizine have the most data and show efficacy, though, clearly, further controlled trials are needed to confirm these data. Adverse effects should be monitored as well. Larger pediatric trials are required prior to widespread use of levetiracetam and sodium valproate. Zonisamide and gabapentin only have one past evaluation each; therefore, additional studies are warranted before recommending these agents for migraine prophylaxis in children.

Table II. Adverse effects of the antiepileptic drugs, based on data presented in trials reviewed

Adverse Effect	VPA	TPM	GBP	LVT	ZNS	Flunarizine	Mg	PB
Dizziness/ataxia	+		+	+				
Tremor	+							
Paresthesia		+				+		
Cognitive dysfunction		+		+		+		+
Somnolence, drowsiness	+	+		+		+		
Sleep disturbance			+					
Fatigue, asthenia	+	+		+		+		
Irritability				+				
Hyperactivity				+				+
Hostile behaviour, aggressivity				+	+			
Nausea, vomiting	+					+		
Diarrhea, soft stools							+	
Increased appetite/weight gain	+					+		
Anorexia/weight loss		+	+			+		
Alopecia	+							
Kidney stones					+			

VPA: valproic acid; TPM: topiramate; GBP: gabapentin; LVT: levetiracetam; ZNS: zonisamide; Mg: magnesium; PB: phenobarbital.

Beside the urgent need to devise well-designed controlled studies dealing with preventive treatment of migraine in children and adolescents with AEDs, we can envisage other future directions. Other AEDs not mentioned above have been reported to show migraine efficacy in a few uncontrolled adult studies; these include tiagabine and lamotrigine, the latter having been reported to be effective for treatment of migraine aura, but not headache. Similarly, some non-conventional AEDs not mentioned above, such as melatonin and vagus nerve stimulation, have also shown promising results in adult studies, and it would be interesting to assess their efficacy in children and adolescents.

Another future direction which might reveal prosperous stems from the fact that, on one part, AEDs such as TPM have shown efficacy in the treatment of adult and pediatric CDH, on another part, preventive treatment with TPM in patients with episodic migraine may reduce the risk of developing chronic forms of headache. These data raise the question whether, in some instances, AEDs could be used in pediatric episodic migraine to prevent such a chronic evolution.

Table III. Dosing and titration of the antiepileptic drugs

Drug	Initial dose	Titration schedule	Target dose
VPA	10 mg/kg/d BID	Increase by 5 mg/kg/d every 2 weeks	14-45 mg/kg/d BID
TPM	15 mg OD	Increase by 15-25 mg every 2 weeks	6 mg/kg/d BID (max. 200 mg/d)
GBP	10 mg/kg/d BID	Increase by 10 mg/kg/d every week	15-30 mg/kg/d BID
LVT	20 mg/kg/d BID	Increase by 5-10 mg/kg/d every week	40 mg/kg/d BID (max. 1,500 mg/d)
ZNS	1 mg/kg/d BID	Increase by 1 mg/kg/d every 2 weeks	5 mg/kg/d BID (max. 12 mg/kg/d)
Flunarizine	5 mg at bedtime	Increase to 10 mg	5-10 mg OD (in adolescents or weight > 25 kg)
Mg	9 mg elemental		Max. 600 mg TID

GBP: gabapentin; LVT: levetiracetam; Mg: magnesium; PB: phenobarbital; TPM: topiramate; VPA: valproic acid; ZNS: zonisamide.

Finally, unravelling the shared neurobiologic mechanisms underlying both migraine and epilepsy cannot but seed fruitful ways tending ultimately to potential therapeutic fertilization. Future studies dealing with the use of AEDS in migraine prevention may well lead to the identification of more selective targets and benefit to both migraine and epilepsy.

References

- Ashrafi MR, Shabanian R, Zamani GR, Mahfelati F. Sodium valproate *versus* propranolol in pediatric migraine prophylaxis. *Eur J Paediatr Neurol* 2005; 9: 333-8.

- Battistella PA, Ruffilli R, Moro R, et al. A placebo-controlled crossover trial of nimodipine in pediatric migraine. *Headache* 1990; 30: 264-8.

- Belman AL, Milazo M, Savatic M, Gabis L. Gabapentin for migraine prophylaxis in children. *Ann Neurol* 2001; 50 (suppl. 1): 109.

- Boccia G, Del Giudice E, Crisanti AF, et al. Functional gastrointestinal disorders in migrainous children: efficacy of flunarizine. *Cephalalgia* 2006; 26: 1214-9.

- Campistol J, Campos J, Casas C, Herranz JL. Topiramate in the prophylactic treatment of migraine in children. *J Child Neurol* 2005; 20: 251-3.

- Caruso JM, Brown WD, Exil G, Gascon GG. The efficacy of divalproex sodium in the prophylactic treatment of children with migraine. *Headache* 2000; 40: 672-6.

- Castellana M, Carini U, Caprici G, Mazzochi B. Calcium entry blockers in the treatment of primary headache in childhood: our experience with flunarizine and nimodipine. In: Lanzi G, Balottin U, Cernibori A, eds. *Headache in Children and Adolescents. Proceedings of the First International Symposium on Headache in Children and Adolescents, 1988 May 19-20, Pavia, Italy*. New York: Elsevier, 1989: 349-52.

- Desmedt LK, Niemegeers CJ, Janssen PA. Anticonvulsive properties of cinnarizine and flunarizine in rats and mice. *Arzneimittelforschung* 1975; 25: 1408-13.

- DeSouza TG, Shahid A, Waran SP. The use of levetiracetam in the prophylactic treatment of migraine headaches in adolescents migraine. *Headache* 2005; 45: 819-20.

- Ferreira J, Garcia N, Pedreira L. Topiramate in pediatric and adolescent migraine patients: a retrospective analysis. *Headache* 2002; 42: 453.

- Fusco C, Pisani F, Capone C, Faienza C. Valproic acid in migraine prophylaxis of young patients. Three new reports. *Acta Biomed* 2002; 73: 47-51.

- Gokhale R, Huttenlocher PR, Brady L, Kirschner BS. Use of barbiturates in the treatment of cyclic vomiting during childhood. *J Pediatr Gastroenterol Nutr* 1997; 25: 64-7. Erratum in: *J Pediatr Gastroenterol Nutr* 1997; 25: 559.

- Hershey AD, Powers SW, Vockell AL, et al. Effectiveness of topiramate in the prevention of childhood headaches. *Headache* 2002; 42: 810-8.

- Kothare SV. Efficacy of flunarizine in the prophylaxis of cyclical vomiting syndrome and abdominal migraine. *Eur J Paediatr Neurol* 2005; 9: 23-6.

- Lakshmi CV, Singhi P, Malhi P, Ray MJ. Topiramate in the prophylaxis of pediatric migraine: a double-blind placebo-controlled trial. *J Child Neurol* 2007; 22: 829-35.

- Lastra Martinez L, Herranz Fernandez J, Arteaga Manjon-Cabez AR. Flunarizina o dihidroergotamina en el tratamiento de la migrana en la infancia. Estudio randomizado de 50 pacientes. *Anales Espanoles de Pediatria* 1990; 32: 213-8.

- Lewis D, Ashwal S, Hershey A, et al. American Academy of Neurology Quality Standards Subcommittee; Practice Committee of the Child Neurology Society. Practice parameter: pharmacological treatment of migraine headache in children and adolescents: report of the American Academy of Neurology Quality Standards Subcommittee and the Practice Committee of the Child Neurology Society. *Neurology* 2004; 63: 2215-24.

- Lewis D, Paradiso E. A double-blind, dose comparison study of topiramate for prophylaxis of basilar-type migraine in children: a pilot study. *Headache* 2007; 47: 1409-17.

- Lütschg J, Vassella F. Behandlung der kindlichen Migräne mit Flunarizin bzw. Propranolol. *Schweiz Med Wochenschr* 1990; 120: 1731-6.

- Mendizabal JE. Extended-release divalproex sodium improves the quality of life of adolescent migraineurs. *Headache* 2002; 42: 327-8.

- Miller GS. Efficacy and safety of levetiracetam in pediatric migraine. *Headache* 2004; 44: 238-43.

- Olmez A, Kose G, Turanli G. Cyclic vomiting with generalized epileptiform discharges responsive to topiramate therapy. *Pediatr Neurol* 2006; 35: 348-51.

- Overweg J, Binnie CD. Flunarizine. In: Dam M, Gram L, eds. *Comprehensive Epileptology*. New York: Raven Press, 1990: 655-64.

- Pakalnis A, Greenberg G, Drake ME Jr, Paolichi J. Pediatric migraine prophylaxis with divalproex. *J Child Neurol* 2001; 16: 731-4.

- Pakalnis A, Kring D. Zonisamide prophylaxis in refractory pediatric headache. *Headache* 2006; 46: 804-7.

- Pakalnis A, Kring D, Meier L. Levetiracetam prophylaxis in pediatric migraine: an open-label study. *Headache* 2007; 47: 427-30.

- Palmer GM, Cameron DJ. Use of intravenous midazolam and clonidine in cyclical vomiting syndrome: a case report. *Paediatr Anaesth* 2005; 15: 68-72. Comment in: *Paediatr Anaesth* 2005; 15: 709-10.

- Pothmann R. Calcium-antagonist flunarizine *vs.* low-dose acetylsalicylic acid in childhood migraine: a double-blind study. *Cephalalgia* 1987a; 7 (suppl. 6): 385-6.

- Pothmann R. Migraneprophylaxe mit Flunarizin und Azetylsalizylsaure. Eine Doppelblindstudie. *Monatsschrift für Kinderheilkunde* 1987b; 135: 646-9.

- Serdaroglu G, Erhan E, Tekgul H, *et al*. Sodium valproate prophylaxis in childhood migraine. *Headache* 2002; 42: 819-22.

- Shaygannejad V, Janghorbani M, Ghorbani A, *et al*. Comparison of the effect of topiramate and sodium valporate in migraine prevention: a randomized blinded crossover study. *Headache* 2006; 46: 642-8.

- Sorge F, Marano E. Flunarizine *vs.* placebo in childhood migraine: a double-blind study. *Cephalalgia* 1985; 5 (suppl. 2): 145-8.

- Sorge F, de Simone R, Marano E, *et al*. Flunarizine in prophylaxis of childhood migraine: a double-blind, placebo-controlled, crossover study. *Cephalalgia* 1988; 8: 1-6.

- Stevenson SB. Epilepsy and migraine headache: is there a connection? *J Pediatr Health Care* 2006; 20: 167-71.

- Tfelt-Hansen P, Block G, Dahlöf C, *et al*. for the International Headache Society Clinical Trials Subcommittee. l. Guidelines for controlled trials of drugs in migraine: second edition. *Cephalalgia* 2000; 20: 765-86.

- Vaisleib II, Neft RA, Schor NF. Role of levetiracetam in prophylaxis of migraine headaches in childhood. *Neurology* 2005; 64: A343.

- Victor S, Ryan S. Drugs for preventing migraine headaches in children. *Cochrane Database System Reviews* 2003; 4: CD 002761.

- Visudtibhan A, Lusawat A, Chiemchanya S, Visudhiphan P. Flunarizine for prophylactic treatment of childhood migraine. *J Med Assoc Thai* 2004; 87: 1466-70.

- Wang F, Van Den Eeden SK, Ackerson LM, *et al*. Oral magnesium oxide prophylaxis of frequent migrainous headache in children: a randomized, double-blind, placebo-controlled trial. *Headache* 2003; 43: 601-10.

- Wasiewski WW. Preventive therapy in pediatric migraine. *J Child Neurol* 2001; 16: 71-8.

- Winner P, Pearlman EM, Linder SL, *et al*. for the Topiramate Pediatric Migraine Study Investigators. Topiramate for migraine prevention in children: a randomized, double-blind, placebo-controlled trial. *Headache* 2005; 45: 1304-12.

- Winner P, Gendolla A, Stayer C, *et al*. Topiramate for migraine prevention in adolescents: a pooled analysis of efficacy and safety. *Headache* 2006; 46: 1503-10.

- Yamane LE, Montenegro MA, Guerreiro MM. Comorbidity headache and epilepsy in childhood. *Neuropediatrics* 2004; 35: 99-102.

- Younkin D. Topiramate in the treatment of pediatric migraine.*Headache* 2002; 42: 456.

Achevé d'imprimer par Corlet, Imprimeur, S.A.
14110 Condé-sur-Noireau
N° d'Imprimeur : 123930 - Dépôt légal : novembre 2009
Imprimé en France